THE PHILOSOPHY OF PUBLIC HEALTH

Public health is a particular area of medical practice that raises a series of philosophical issues that require urgent discussion. The philosophy of public health includes metaphysical questions such as, what do we mean by 'public' in public health? How ought we to conceptualise the idea of 'populations'? Are they merely aggregations of individuals? It also includes epistemological questions such as, what methods are most appropriate for thinking about public health? How do empirical and normative issues relate to each other? Controversial ethical, political and social issues, including those relating to vaccinations, the threat of pandemics and possible restrictions to individual liberties, public health research, screening and obesity policy should also be considered. This volume includes a diverse set of papers exploring a number of the most important theoretical and practical issues that arise across the whole field of the philosophy of public health.

The Philosophy of Public Health

Edited by

ANGUS DAWSON
Keele University, UK

ASHGATE

Published by
Ashgate Publishing Limited
Wey Court East
Union Road
Farnham
Surrey, GU9 7PT
England

Ashgate Publishing Company
Suite 420
101 Cherry Street
Burlington
VT 05401-4405
USA

www.ashgate.com

British Library Cataloguing in Publication Data
The philosophy of public health
1. Public health – Philosophy
I. Dawson, Angus
362.1'01

Library of Congress Cataloging-in-Publication Data
Dawson, Angus.
The philosophy of public health / Angus Dawson.
p. cm.
ISBN 978-0-7546-6043-9 (hardcover : alk. paper)
1. Public health–Philosophy. I. Title.

RA427.D39 2008
362.101–dc22

2008044321

ISBN 978 0 7546 6043 9
EISBN 978-0-7546-9357-4

Mixed Sources
Product group from well-managed forests and other controlled sources
www.fsc.org Cert no. SGS-COC-2482
© 1996 Forest Stewardship Council
FSC

Printe
TJ Inte

Contents

List of Figures and Table

Figures

Table

Acknowledgments

The papers in this edited collection were all originally presented at the annual conference of the Society for Applied Philosophy, held in Manchester, UK, 30 June-2 July 2006, on the theme of 'The Philosophy of Public Health'. Thanks to all of the speakers, respondents and chairs that helped to make the conference such a successful event. Thanks also to the executive committee of the Society for Applied Philosophy for asking me to organize the conference, especially Gordon Graham and David Archard. I'd also like to thank Richard Ashcroft, Ruth Chadwick and Marcel Verweij, for the help they gave me at different times in relation to this event; all at Chancellors, Manchester University for the smooth running of the conference; and Jon Cameron for all of his excellent work behind the scenes. More recent thanks go to Trevor King and Louise Ennis for their help in preparing the manuscript for publication, and the Centre for Ethics, University of Toronto, for providing a wonderful environment for writing. Thanks also to Bev Sykes for work on the proofs and the index. Finally, thanks go to all at Ashgate, especially Sarah Charters, Rachel Lynch, Anne Keirby and Paul Coulam for their patience.

Chapter 1
Introduction: the Philosophy of Public Health

Angus Dawson
Keele University, UK

1. A Philosophy of Public Health

In this chapter I seek to introduce the other chapters in this volume, but also to provide some context and content for the idea of a 'philosophy of public health'. A logical place to start is with the question: what is a philosophy of public health? However, to answer this broad question we have to address two prior sub-questions about the nature of both 'philosophy' and 'public health'. So, let us begin with what we mean by 'philosophy'.

Is it possible to defend a particular definition of 'philosophy'? It is in fact very difficult to do so, as the meaning and scope of philosophy is itself a philosophical issue, often open to rancorous debate. However, there are perhaps three main ways to offer such a definition. I will call these three: the 'methodology' approach, the 'content' approach, and the 'attitude' approach. First, the advocates of the methodology approach argue that philosophy differs from other disciplines in that it requires the use of a particular methodology. Candidates for the relevant methodology are legion, but a focus on analysis and argument is central (at least within the Anglo-American philosophical tradition). The second 'content' approach suggests that philosophy has a particular traditional set of concerns or subjects. Examples of this approach might include a focus on asking (and attempting to answer) fundamental questions about ourselves and our world, or in a more mundane form, philosophy is just held to be a list of sub-disciplines (e.g. ethics, metaphysics, epistemology and aesthetics etc.). The third approach holds that philosophy is not so much a method or subject, but more of an attitude (involving, for example, the development of a questioning, sceptical nature). For our purposes here we do not need to take any strong line in adopting any one particular account. In fact, these three views are not strictly mutually exclusive, and they may be combined in different ways. One additional perspective, and a possible way to offer a neat unity, might be to return to the etymological roots of philosophy and look towards the idea of philosophy as loving or seeking wisdom. Certainly, pursuing what is required by some accounts of the concept of 'wisdom' will keep us rather busy.[1] Perhaps it is best to adopt a more pragmatic definition, one that at least nods towards all of the above approaches. Such a view would see philosophy as being concerned with the underlying assumptions that lie behind our concepts, perspectives and social practices.

Secondly, we will need to have some working definition of what we mean when we talk about 'public health'. This again is harder than it might seem, as the term is subject to much disagreement and debate in the literature.[2] We might begin by stipulating public health as being everything that public health policy makers and practitioners do. However, this looks too imprecise in that it is neither a necessary nor sufficient condition for public health: other people can contribute to public health and public health professionals may possibly act in contravention of public health at times. This means we are inevitably driven to adopt a more conceptual approach in an attempt to try and pick out the key features of public health. Many of the definitions focus on two core elements to (at least paradigm cases of) public health activity: first, a focus on the health of the 'public' as the object of action (in the sense of a group or population) and, second, that the mode of intervention requires action and participation by many people (often through the coordinated action of government or its representatives).[3] Public health, then, requires knowledge about harms to health at a population level (hence the requirement for particular methodologies, such as epidemiology) and seeks to remove them (often through collective participation).

So can we now get any clearer about what a philosophy of public health might be? Is there such a thing? Certainly, there is no thriving discipline answering to this name. There are no departments, chairs, or research programmes named after or working on this topic; and the literature explicitly focused on this 'topic' is remarkably small. In fact I have only been able to find six papers with philosophy of public health in the title. The earliest piece by Julius Prince (1958) is interested in the idea of what he termed a 'public philosophy' for public health.[4] However, this is really an early call for community engagement, as a means of facilitating the implementation of public health policy. While his real interest is in the practical requirement to engage with public officials on the grounds of efficiency, he also sees it as being important in a political sense to consult and engage with the public when formulating and implementing public health policy in a democracy. Kozo Tatara's (2002) more recent paper is not really about philosophy in the relevant

---

1 See, for example, S. Ryan. (2007) 'Wisdom'. *Stanford Encyclopedia of Philosophy*. Stanford: Stanford University Press. See: http://plato.stanford.edu/entries/wisdom/ (accessed January 2008).

2 M. Verweij and A. Dawson. (2007) 'The meaning of "public" in "public health"'. In A. Dawson and M. Verweij (eds). (2007) *Ethics, Prevention and Public Health*. Oxford: Oxford University Press.

3 Again, see Verweij and Dawson (2007).

4 J.S. Prince (1958) 'A public philosophy in public health'. *American Journal of Public Health*. 48/7: 903-12.

sense.[5] He is more interested in philosophy in the sense of popular usage: here philosophy is seen as the way that you might approach a topic. Such a view may be incorporated into the more technical philosophy of public health (e.g. how *ought* we to approach public health?), but need not be. The three papers to really address the true core issues relating to the philosophy of public health are those by van der Maesen and Nijhuis[6] [7] and Douglas Weed.[8] Both of these sets of authors agree on the need to critique and think through the assumptions behind public health practice, policy and research methods. They jointly focus on the need to consider and debate the role of key ideas within public health (such as notions of causality and evidence, the relationship between population and individual benefit and harm, and the meaning of central concepts such as those of 'public' and 'health'). Weed is particularly clear in his call for a general philosophy of public health, one that will attend to the full range of ontological, epistemic and ethical aspects that arise in the contemplation of what public health is and does. Lastly, Beauchamp's chapter (1995) in the *Encyclopedia of Bioethics* is an interesting addition to the literature, as he is not so much calling for a philosophy of public health, as attempting to develop the beginnings of such an account.[9] Beauchamp's starting point is very much with trying to fill out what he takes to be the central concepts in public health, such as that of 'community' and to use this to argue that a view of public health built upon such a tradition will be very different from one focused on individuals and their behaviour.[10]

However, despite this relative neglect in the literature, I want to claim that there is certainly something that we can coherently call a 'philosophy of public health' in two senses. Firstly, even if there is little current literature, a philosophy of public health certainly exists as an area of discourse or a topic, in the same way that there is a philosophy of physics, biology or medicine. Of course, it is not so developed as these other examples, but there is no *a priori* reason why it should not be so in the future. This is the topic that is discussed by van der Maesen and Nijhuis, Weed and Beauchamp. It will be an important part of the job of this discipline to define

---

[5] K. Tatara. 'Philosophy of public health'. *Journal of Public Health Medicine*. 24/1: 11-15.

[6] H.G.J. Nijhuis and L.J.G. van der Maesen (1994) 'The philosophical foundations of public health: an invitation to debate'. *Journal of Epidemiology and Community Health*. 48: 1-3.

[7] L.J.G. van der Maesen and H.G.J. Nijhuis (2000) 'Continuing the debate on the philosophy of modern public health: social quality as a point of reference'. *Journal of Epidemiology and Community Health*. 54: 134-142.

[8] D.L. Weed (1999) 'Towards a philosophy of public health'. *Journal of Epidemiology and Community Health*. 53: 99-104.

[9] D.E. Beauchamp. (1995) 'Philosophy of public health'. In: W.T. Reich (ed.) *Encyclopedia of Bioethics*. New York: Simon and Schuster Macmillan.

[10] D.E. Beauchamp (1985) 'Community: the neglected tradition of public health'. *Hastings Center Report*. 15: 28-36.

its specific place and content and its relationship to other areas of discourse, such as the philosophy of medicine. Secondly, public health activity (in terms of both policy and practice) is full of issues crying out for more philosophical critique and discussion as all of the authors above suggest. Many of the different sub-branches of philosophy (ethics, epistemology, metaphysics, social and political philosophy, even aesthetics) are clearly relevant to discussion about such topics as the meaning, nature and role of statistical inferences, the contribution to be made by social science methods to public health, the meaning of cause and effect in public health, the relative roles of physiological and environmental factors in the genesis of medical conditions and the meaning of concepts such as harm, risk and prevention. There is no reason why these two different tracks cannot be pursued at the same time. However, the latter approach of focusing on specific issues and concepts will be the one where we are likely to see the most progress in the near future. The grander vision of a general and unified philosophy of public health may be some way off.

2. The Richness and Diversity of Philosophies of Public Health

The papers in this volume illustrate the wide range of topics, methods and approaches that can be employed in arguments, and the richness and diversity of themes that can be explored from the perspective of the philosophy of public health.

Robyn Martin discusses the function of the law in public health. She concentrates in this chapter on outlining and discussing two different roles for law in relation to public health. The first is the contribution that law can make as a tool to assist the implementation of public health policy, and the second, is the role of law in relation to public health ethics through the legal enforcement of rights. In relation to the first role she concentrates on discussing three methods: legislation, criminal law, and law as a mechanism for enforcing public attitudes. Each of these methods demonstrates different advantages and problems. In essence law is a powerful tool, in that individuals can be monitored, investigated and have various freedoms curtailed and removed. However, law arising from statute is a rather crude instrument in that it tends to reflect the scientific beliefs and values of the time it was created. This means it can be inappropriate in two ways (being concerned with issues that are now irrelevant and having no means to respond to new and previously unimagined threats). Old laws are bent to fit new situations, whereas new laws can be dangerously wide. We need to be clear about what our public health aims are, so that we can then try and shape the law to attain those ends. However, we need to realize that the law, whilst useful, is not always the answer: it can also create its own problems. This point is well illustrated by the second issue that Martin discusses, namely the role of law in relation to the enforcement of rights. The law, through tort action and the application of human rights legislation can act as an important tool for the protection of individuals. However, in relation to public health, the use of such powers may result in a detrimental impact to the public's health, even whilst protecting individuals.

In her chapter, 'Luck, Risk and Prevention', Katherine King explores what taking the idea of prevention seriously might mean for theories of distributive justice. She begins by distinguishing between the cases of compensation for existing disadvantage and that of preventing future disadvantage (although it quickly becomes apparent that in real life, a clear distinction is often impossible to draw). King chooses to focus her discussion on Dworkin's account of luck egalitarianism, because the prevention (or reduction in the possibility) of some harm is likely to increase opportunity. She argues, convincingly, that the resources of Dworkin's theory cannot sufficiently take into account the idea of prevention, as the account of option and brute luck are inadequate as a means of capturing this concept. She proposes that we adopt the idea of risk rather than luck for two reasons. First, it is better able to capture the future-directedness of prevention and, second, the idea of risk can be seen as a feature of a group or population that an individual belongs to, not just as something individual-related. This approach is an interesting addition to the literature on luck-egalitarianism and of direct interest to justice concerns in public health.

Patricia Illingworth's discussion of social capital is innovatory because she takes a concept that originated in sociology and public policy literature and argues that it can also be understood as a normative concept, and should therefore be of interest to those working on ethical and political issues in public health. Her discussion begins with an analysis of the concept, with a focus on the work of Robert Putnam in particular. Social capital is held to be vital for the possibility of social activity, particularly because of its relation to trust and reciprocity, therefore it is held by many to be a necessary requirement for effective public health activity. Illingworth argues that, despite the vagueness of the concept, it should be seen to be an ethical concept because it is something that we *ought* to pursue both for its own sake, but also, perhaps more importantly for what it, in turn, enables. It is a concept that requires social relationships with others for its existence: it cannot be created by a single person and it imposes obligations upon others. This in turn, according to Illingworth, suggests that the duty to cultivate social capital falls upon both individuals and institutions (although this will only be a *prima facie* duty, so it will have to be traded against other important moral considerations). Social capital, it is argued, has the potential to contribute to discussions about global justice as well as more 'local' concerns about how individuals relate to each other in their immediate communities. It will certainly be interesting to see how the discussion of social capital, and its implications for our normative commitments, develop over the coming years.

Onyebuchi Arah's chapter shifts the discussion from the legal, social, political and ethical, to the issue of what public health is and how we ought to evaluate the performance of public health activities. He argues that we should think of public health as involving two aspects: the health of the public (in the sense of the aggregative population, which he calls the *ends* perspective) and the public of health (which he terms the *means* perspective). Public health activity will have to measure (and be evaluated in terms of) both of these aspects. Current attempts to measure public health performance seem inadequate for this task. Arah argues that the success of public health needs to be measured in terms of the provision and distribution of opportunities as well as the actual health attainments of individuals within a population. He suggests that this approach may reduce some of the tension in normative discussions in relation to the relative weight to be assigned to the individual and the collective within a framework of public health ethics.

In his chapter, Søren Holm argues that whilst a globalized bioethics might well be a legitimate goal, we need to take care about how we approach this end. The danger is that we just apply our 'local' ethical approach to the globe (assuming that this is the correct approach, and ignoring any contentious features in such an application) or we just apply what we take to be a 'consensus' view, failing to realize the role of power in the very fact that a particular approach is held to be the consensus. Holm argues that we cannot just take the easy route to globalized bioethics through an adoption of human rights or a particular institutional framework or set of procedures. He argues that even a principle such as respect for autonomy, that has been so central to so many discussions in Western bioethics, can be inappropriately 'globalized'.

Gillian Brock focuses her chapter on the impact of the migration of healthcare workers from the developing world to the developed world. She outlines the scale of the problem (with many countries now losing workers faster than they can train them) before using this example to ask a more general question about the obligations that the developed world has to the populations affected. Does the migration of such staff have an impact upon health? Undoubtedly. The developing world is not only losing staff to the developed world, but it is in effect subsidizing the healthcare of the developed world. Various Codes of Practice for recruitment policies are considered and found wanting in their focus on voluntariness and their limited application to only certain countries, resulting in a lack of attention to the scale of the consequences for populations in the developing world. The result of Brock's argument is a positive claim for compensation for past wrongs, perhaps with a focus on investment in both healthcare training and the healthcare systems of the developing world. Brock argues that it is the employing institutions that should bear the compensation costs.

Paula Boddington subjects Shared Responsibility Agreements (SRAs) to a critical review. She focuses on their use in Australia, particularly in relation to welfare policy for aboriginal populations. She systematically and carefully reviews the discussions that have taken place over these agreements. However, her argument is that whatever the quality of these other objections, SRAs are too simplistic, in that they fail to capture the complexity of the causal processes that have created the situations addressed. Responsibility for past 'failures' tends to focus on the actions of individuals or particular communities, ignoring historical and societal factors, and underplaying or discounting the contribution of inequalities and injustices such as racism. In addition, Boddington argues that the frequent use of the word 'responsibility' in relation to SRAs tends to ignore the important difference between causal responsibility (the contribution made) and the moral responsibility for addressing the problem (as it exists). Exactly who is responsible and obligated to act is often left vague. Boddington focuses on a particular agreement, the first Mulan Agreement, to bring out many of the issues relating to the complexity of causation in such cases.

Kalle Grill discusses paternalism in public health policy, focusing on the issue of the safety of consumer products. He argues that when we talk of paternalism we need to take care that we are identifying the right reason behind an action, as only some of the reasons will count as paternalistic. In regard to product safety regulation, Grill argues that even if some will welcome product safety laws, there are good reasons to think that some will not. Where such interference in free choice is unwelcome, and justified by appeal to the good of the person, paternalism may exist. The focus on reasons for the action allows us to consider whether the action really is paternalistic. The mere accusation of paternalism should not be enough to tell against a public health policy. More exploration of the reasons behind the policy is required in any evaluation of both the claim of paternalism and more general concerns about the justifiability of the action.

Niels Nijsingh discusses an important ethical issue arising from new developments in neonatal screening programmes. The problem concerns the ability to screen for multiple disorders so quickly and easily with new technologies, and the fact that it is not always easy to decide to screen for a particular disorder, as the result of one test might disclose information about another disorder. He considers just such a case and what it might mean to have an autonomous right to the information supplied by the test. He argues that it makes no sense to construe decisions about such cases as being about choosing information, although parents can of course give consent for their child to undergo screening. This is because of the paradox of information provision in such cases: information is only of interest if it is positive, but by asking if someone wants to know, you are already suggesting what the outcome is.

Benjamin and Lauren Hale's interdisciplinary chapter on issues relating to sleep is a stimulating and original discussion of a neglected issue. They contrast two different models for conceptualizing how we could think about sleep (the linear and curvilinear models) and suggest that the latter is a better fit with the empirical evidence. They also present two different models for framing the way that we think about sleep (the 'choice view' and the 'autonomy view'). They argue that the latter is to be preferred because of the way that autonomy is tied to the idea of self-determination and the setting and fulfilling of life projects. The optimal amount of sleep is a necessary requirement not just for health, but also for the enhancement of autonomy (in this sense). This in turn has implications for public health activities, in that the focus of policy and practice should be on a much wider frame of considerations than merely that of sleep.

In her chapter, Catherine Womack begins to review a core set of issues relating to obesity policy and how they ought to be conceptualized and addressed. Like the previous chapter, this one explores a set of philosophical issues arising from a discussion of empirical literature. Womack argues that the normative discussion in relation to obesity needs to be radically reevaluated as many researchers look for ways to bring about individual behaviour change in relation to diet and exercise. Womack suggests that this will prove to be inadequate because we already have good evidence that such interventions will prove ineffective. She argues that we need to think about innovative collective interventions as a means to contribute to individual behaviour change. This chapter serves as a good example of the kind of deeper reflection we need in relation to empirical evidence to allow paradigm shifts in public policy.

Marcel Verweij discusses a set of ethical issues related to vaccination research and policy, where there is an interest in reducing the number of doses from the recommended and previously researched schedule (for reasons of cost or vaccine shortage). He illustrates his discussion by using the example of debates about routine pneumococcal vaccination for young children in the Netherlands. For reasons of cost, there was the possibility of instituting a three dose schedule instead of the usual four doses. However, this raised the issue about the effectiveness of such a reduced schedule. A randomized clinical trial could be used to determine the answer using one of two models, either 3 doses verses 4 doses or 3 doses versus placebo. The first option was judged to be infeasible because of the numbers of participants and the time needed to provide a statistically significant answer. However, the second option for a trial (3 doses versus placebo) looked problematic for ethical reasons, as it was held that researchers involved in the trial could not be in equipoise, as given the original 4 dose trial it was already clear that 3 doses would be better than placebo. Verweij explores reasons to think that equipoise might be less relevant in such cases than first thought. For example, such a vaccine trial would be focused on a preventive intervention involving healthy subjects, rather than patients requiring treatment, so it is unclear how the special duty of beneficence owed by physicians towards their patients will apply. Other considerations relating to justice might also be relevant, although Verweij argues that the background level of public health provision within a society may be relevant to the justification of such trials. This chapter is an interesting illustration of how ethical, policy and methodological issues in public health are all interwoven.

In their chapter, Francis et al. provide a historical analysis of the development of bioethics and use this to argue that there has been a relative neglect of discussions of the ethical issues relating to both infectious disease in particular, but also the wider field of public health in general. Much of this focus is traced to the political drive of much early bioethics work, drawing upon the civil rights traditions, and focusing on such issues as informed consent and privacy. They suggest that the opportunity for a reassessment provided by the emergence of the HIV epidemic was missed, and that many of the discussions of HIV ignored the fact it was an infectious disease. This 'exceptionalism' was encouraged by both the (mainly sexual) mode of transmission and the strong focus right from the outset (at least in the developing world) upon the need to protect the important civil liberties of marginalized groups in society. Since the emergence of HIV, Francis et al. point to an important contrasting trend that draws upon public health activities and traditions. They argue that discussions in the literature on this topic have been invigorated by a focus on the idea of the importance of population health, an increasing interest by many in health at the global level and development issues and public health practitioners' own willingness and enthusiasm for reflecting upon and critiquing their own values and practice. They argue that it is now time to draw these traditions more closely together, and they offer the idea of looking at those carrying infectious disease as being both victim and vector, that is as both the faultless sufferer from disease as well as the potential agent for infecting others.

In her chapter, Charlotte Paul provides a stimulating argument for public health traditions to provide a framework for critically addressing some aspects of preventive public health activity. She discusses HIV prevention and the actual (and future potential) role of preventive activities focused on partner reduction as a means of reducing HIV transmission. Lowering the number of sexual partners certainly provides greater protection for the individual and the population. However, policies focused on seeking to change people's behaviour in this regard have been subject to vociferous criticism. There is a great reluctance to talk about how others should behave, especially in relation to sexual matters, even by those working to reduce HIV. She argues that even increasing sexual activity by just a single partner can be demonstrated to have a dramatic effect on everyone's risk of being infected with HIV within a population. Paul discusses the empirical evidence of success in partner reduction campaigns in Uganda and Botswana and suggests that if we are serious in seeking to reduce risks of transmission, then we must focus on norms and explore different means for changing them. Paul focuses on what she terms 'common good arguments', such as the common interest in protecting one's community from HIV transmission. She uses the work of Geoffrey Rose, now a public health classic, to illustrate the way that individual behaviour can have an impact upon population health (and *vice versa*). Such arguments are a rich source for the future development of arguments in public health ethics.

Finally, in his chapter Martin Wilkinson explores the apparent conflict between (at least some) rights (such as the right to liberty, bodily integrity, privacy etc.) and public health activities focused on the protection of the public from potential harm. He discusses the possible grounds for compulsory treatment, detention and preventive activities, and explores three different possible justifications for such compulsion. The first one is that the relevant rights are not absolute and can be overridden (in at least some circumstances). Second, that other people's rights (e.g. not to be infected) are important, and that something like a right to self-defence can be invoked. Third, that given the nature of the transmission of infectious diseases, a focus on individual rights will produce collective action problems. Wilkinson argues that the first justification is problematic due to the difficulties in justifying any non-arbitrary thresholds for interventions and calculating the relevant probabilities of harm. He suggests that the second is more promising, as the idea of self-defence provides a more robust objection than focusing on other kinds of overriding rights. However, it is the third justification that is perhaps the strongest, in that if we can make sense of a coherent notion of the relevant collective issues, we might be able to use this as a means to stave off the problematic outcomes (for the collective) that can be produced through respecting certain individual actions.

3. A Philosophy of Public Health?

Many of these papers concentrate on ethical issues in public health practice, and this is perhaps the strongest area of a developing philosophy of public health. Public health ethics is a rapidly growing area of applied ethics in its own right. However, virtually all of these papers appeal to empirical claims or empirical evidence during the course of their arguments. Where such evidence is considered, other aspects of a philosophy of public health cannot be avoided. The epistemic and metaphysical issues necessary to thinking through how we should discuss issues relating to populations and groups rather than individuals certainly require more work. As I suggested above, there is not really any such thing as a philosophy of public health in terms of a substantive discipline, so it is no surprise that this volume is far from being the last word on this topic. However, this edited collection illustrates the fact that there are important issues to be explored here, and it will be exciting to see how this field develops in the future. Perhaps one day there really will be a philosophy of public health.

Chapter 2
The Role of Law in Public Health

Robyn Martin
Hertfordshire University, UK and Chinese University of Hong Kong

Is there anything which law can contribute to the improvement of public health? We already have a profession of public health practitioners from a wide range of disciplines, epidemiologists, statisticians, doctors, sociologists, research scientists and health economists, doing sterling work to protect us from communicable and non-communicable disease. We also have a developing scholarship on public health ethics, not yet as sophisticated and refined as medical ethics, but with the potential to provide a useful framework for good public health practice. Is there any added value in introducing law as yet another form of public health governance?

I would argue that there are two potential roles of law in public health. One role is to contribute to the work that public health professionals do; that is to provide tools which can be used to protect populations from communicable and non-communicable diseases. The other role is to contribute to the work that ethics does; that is to assist in the provision of a framework for good public health practice.

In order to examine whether law can contribute anything useful in relation to either of these roles, I will consider two recognized functions of law, law as a means of social control as a public health tool, and law as a protector of rights as a contribution to the framework of good public health practice. My discussion will focus mainly on the laws of England and Wales, but for reasons which I will later explain, much of what I will say will have resonance for readers from other jurisdictions.

Law and Social Control as a Tool for Public Health Professionals

Jurisprudential debate around law's empire over the last three hundred years or so suggests that one of the most important functions of law is the maintenance of social order.[1] Of course there are other means of social control such as politics, economics, custom, religion, morals and systems of morals, which we call ethics. None of these operate independently. Ethics and law for example overlap, and good law should be underpinned by ethics. But law has different objectives to

---

[1] See for example the work of Roscoe Pound, in particular *Social Control Through Law* (New Brunswick, NJ and London: Transaction Publishers, 1997).

ethics, and different objectives to other forms of societal governance such as economics or politics.

The primary purpose of ethics, and indeed of politics and even economics, can be said to assess the value of policies, interventions and behaviours, so as to enable us to formulate criteria for measuring the relative value of particular interests. Law goes one stage further, and having made an assessment of values, it provides mechanisms for making those values effective. Law has at its disposal tools such as legislation, the judicial process and regulatory systems which enable both public bodies and policy makers to ensure that their value-based policies and interventions are carried out.

Law is an imperfect vehicle for ensuring that democratic values are upheld. There are some things that law does quite well, and others where law is too clumsy, too slow, too confrontational and too heavy a hand to give effect to values. And it is often the case that the values which law seeks to enforce are themselves flawed, flawed in the sense that they are based on insufficient evidence, flawed in that they represent the values of particular powerful sections of society, or flawed in that they cannot be justified by principles of ethics or human rights. Such concerns, as we shall see, have particular application to our public health law.

Custom, religion and moral systems also come with sanctions for dealing with those who disobey. But law has a longer, and stronger, arm. Law has a longer arm in that it can reach those who do not subscribe to a customary norm or a religious principle or a system of morals. Sanctions such as social approbation or exclusion only work against persons who would feel threatened by unpopularity or exclusion. Law applies to everyone, whether they believe in the power of the state or not, whether they subscribe to the values underpinning law or not. Law has a stronger arm in that it has enforcement mechanisms not available to other social regulators. Law can exert physical coercion. Law endows public bodies and individuals with the power, right or duty to exercise physical force to ensure that a law is obeyed. Law determines who may exercise physical coercion as a socially recognized privilege or right and allocates authority to such persons. There are other effective mechanisms at law's disposal—fines, awards of damages, injunctions to prevent behaviour, declarations through the process of judicial review to insist that public bodies behave in certain ways, and systems of licensing which can make behaviour a condition of particular desirable goods.

So what legal tools of social control are available to protect public health? I will examine three: public health legislation, the criminal law, and law as a dictator of public attitudes.

Public Health Legislation

The core statutory public health law in England and Wales can be found in the *Public Health (Control of Disease) Act 1984* and the subsidiary *Public Health (Infectious Diseases) Regulations 1988*. We must not be fooled by the dates of the legislation. The 1984 Act is little more than a consolidation of old laws, and our public health statutory framework goes back to the late nineteenth century.

The time of framing of laws is significant because laws represent the value systems of the society at the time at which the laws are made. Custom and religion and systems of morals can evolve and adapt with changing culture, but laws in statutory form remain set in stone, and attempts by the courts to interpret laws so that they reflect contemporary values are hampered by rules of statutory interpretation. Rules of statutory interpretation require that courts give effect to the intention of the statute. It is not the role of the courts to amend the statute because to do so would be to make new law, and that is the responsibility of elected parliament.

At the time when our public health law was first drafted, the underlying philosophies, reflecting contemporary cultural values, were those of utilitarianism and communitarianism. Public health was utilitarian in that it operated to achieve the greatest good for the greatest number, and was not particularly concerned with the health consequences for individuals. It was communitarian in that it assumed that rights and privileges of the individual could be sacrificed if it was necessary to do so for the public good.

The chief architect of our public health legislation was not a doctor but a lawyer, Edwin Chadwick. His inquiry into the state of public health was based on science which at the time understood disease to be transmitted by miasma wafting from sources such as cesspits, unclean water and drains. He concluded that the chief cause of public health harms was unsanitary conditions and as a consequence public health law was framed to focus on control of unsanitary sources of disease. Because the framing of the legislation was the work of a lawyer with little input from the other professions, it was a traditional legal device that was adapted to serve a public health purpose, in particular the device of the statutory nuisance. By categorizing a disease source such as a drain or an unsanitary building as a legal nuisance, then particular legal tools come into play, including powers of control, exclusion, monitoring and licensing. The Act specified a list of diseases which it called 'notifiable diseases', and any recognized source of a notifiable disease was categorized as a nuisance.

Edwin Chadwick's approach to public health law was to have influence around the world. Because of its early leadership in the industrial revolution, Britain faced the public health consequences of industry, pollution, large scale factories and urbanization before most other nations, and it was these problems which necessitated the first public health laws. Not only were the early public health acts transported around the network of British colonies,[2] but also other states seeking to introduce public health controls looked to British law for guidance.

---

2 See C. Reynolds, *Public Health Law and Regulation* (Annondale, NSW: The Federation Press, 2004).

Even countries as culturally and geographically distant as Japan[3], have a public health legal framework closely modelled on British law.

Chadwick's *Public Health Act 1875*, which forms the basis of the 1984 Act, introduced a range of enforcement mechanisms in relation to public health nuisances.

1. The first mechanism was the imposition on public health officials of public health duties. In relation to notifiable diseases, and only those diseases, medical practitioners have statutory duties for the reporting of disease, but also in relation to activities such as the burial of dead bodies and screening of canal boats. Those same duties exist in our current legislation, and the list of notifiable diseases continues to reflect nineteenth-century health concerns (smallpox, cholera, yellow fever), and does not include contemporary health threats such as SARS, human pandemic influenza or non-communicable diseases.
2. The second mechanism introduced by the legislation was statutory powers, particularly compulsory powers such as powers of investigation, forcible removal, and powers of closure. Powers were again linked to the declaration of a disease as a notifiable disease. These powers worked reasonably effectively in relation to drains, wells, cesspits and buildings. But as medical science progressed it came to be realized that it was not miasma but germs which were the cause of disease spread, and that people, like cesspits and drains, could be sources of disease transmission. Rather than create new law to reflect new medical science, the old law was adapted such that people were brought into the nuisance regime.

   Powers were created such that a person, who was infected with disease, or a possible carrier of disease, was categorized as a nuisance and made subject to similar powers to those applied to places. So such a person would be subject to powers of investigation in the form of compulsory medical examination and duties of reporting, powers of exclusion from school, work or the home, and powers of removal in the form of compulsory isolation or quarantine. Consistent with public attitudes at the time, law was framed on a 'them and us' approach, in that law worked to build walls around healthy people to keep them safe from transmission of infection from people who might be possible sources of disease. This same philosophy continues to characterize infectious disease law in most jurisdictions.

   The original public health legislation has gone through several stages of consolidation and minor reform over the years, but the underlying premises have not been questioned. Changing social attitudes to the balance between public good and individual rights have not been reflected in reform. However one more powerful interest did prompt the removal of powers

[3] See K. Tatara, 'Philosophy of public health: lessons from its history in England', *Journal of Public Health Medicine*, 24/1 (2002): 11-15.

of quarantine[4] from our legislation, in the interests of trade. It was realized that quarantine of large numbers of persons who had been in contact with a sufferer of disease, especially in relation to persons on board ships coming from trade ports in Asia, Africa and the Americas, was having a detrimental effect on British trading capacity. All powers of quarantine were removed, and current legislation in England and Wales does not authorize quarantine in relation to any disease.

3. The third mechanism introduced by the 1875 Act is the creation of public health offences in relation to health behaviours. The 1984 legislation continues to list a string of offences for which there are sanctions of fines and possibly imprisonment. If a person is suffering from a notifiable disease it is an offence to travel on public transport, an offence to take washing to a laundry, an offence to return library books, an offence if the landlord or occupier of the house does not disinfect the house, an offence to expose others to risk of disease. Those offences remain in our current legislation, although in many cases there is now no evidence base for the offences. A recent systematic review, for example, found that there was absolutely no disease risk created by a person suffering from disease returning a book to a library.[5]
4. Perhaps the most interesting of these offences are the offences relating to exposing others to risk of disease. If a person is suffering from a notifiable disease and exposes another to risk of infection by his presence or by his conduct, in a street, public place, place of entertainment, club, hotel, inn or shop, he commits an offence under the *Public Health Act*.[6] Indeed a person who has care of another who is infected with disease, and allows the infected person to expose others to disease, commits an offence. These offences appear to have been used only rarely, with the occasional prosecution against someone with tuberculosis who ventured into a public place.[7] Although the offences remained on the statute books, it came to be thought sufficiently discordant with our cultural attitudes to health to prosecute someone for passing on a disease to another. But as we shall see, there has been some movement on those attitudes.

In my discussion of public health legislation I have so far omitted to mention a new piece of legislation which, although it was not framed as a piece of public health legislation, will give the state wide ranging powers in the case of major

---

4 Quarantine is the isolation of persons who are not themselves infected but who have been exposed to a person infected with a communicable disease.

5 R.L. Atenstaedt, 'Does danger lurk in the library?', *Public Health*, 120/8 (2006): 776-7.

6 *Public Health Act (Control of Disease) 1984*, Sections 33 and 34.

7 See R. Martin and L. Johnson, *Law and the Public Dimension of Health* (London: Cavendish Press, 2001): Chapter 3.

public health threats. The *Civil Contingencies Act 2004* was designed to give the state powers in cases of bioterrorism, but it is framed sufficiently broadly to cover any event which can be categorized as an emergency and which threatens damage to human welfare. Many other states have begun to enact similar emergency powers legislation in response to the threat of terrorist attack, but as with the *Civil Contingencies Act*, such legislation is generally worded so as apply beyond terrorism to public emergencies which might include public health threats. These emergency powers may well override or come into conflict with existing public health powers, and it is not clear how such conflict will be resolved.

The *Civil Contingencies Act* allows the passing of regulations to bring into play a wide range of emergency powers and could authorize for example wide-scale isolation and quarantine. No such regulations have yet been passed. While the broad range of possible powers might be useful in the short term if there were to be a sudden and widespread invasion of a dangerous communicable disease, the Act's limitation to situations of emergency means that it *should* have no application to long term, chronic health concerns which are the daily stuff of public health practice. However government commentary on public health appears to presuppose that the *Civil Contingencies Act* will serve to fill the gaps left by our outdated public health legislation.

Criminal Law

The second legal means of social control is the use of criminal law, and I will consider one example in the context of public health.

Recently, another old piece of legislation, the *Offences Against the Person Act 1861*, has been used with consequences for public health, to criminalize harmful public health behaviours. The *Offences Against the Person Act* has never purported to be a public health law statute. It is a criminal law statute designed to protect the public against criminal behaviour, and with the objectives of punishment of persons who behave in anti-social ways and deterrence of anti-social behaviour.

The statute makes it an offence recklessly to cause grievous bodily harm.[8] Several persons in England and Wales, both men and women, have been convicted of recklessly causing grievous bodily harm in that, knowing they were HIV positive, they had sexual intercourse with another without notifying the sexual partner of their HIV status.[9] Similar prosecutions have taken place in Scotland, Australia, USA and Canada, and some US states have specific statutory offences in relation to reckless transmission of AIDS.[10] It is perhaps not irrelevant that the majority of prosecutions in the United Kingdom have been against persons

8 *The Offences Against the Person Act 1861*, Section 20.

9 For example *R v Mohammed Dica* [2004] 3 WLR 213, *R v Feston Konzani* [2005] 2 Cr App R 14.

10 UNAIDS, *Criminal Law, Public Health and HIV Transmission* (Geneva: UNAIDS, 2002).

of African origin. It is also interesting that the majority of prosecutions so far have been in relation to heterosexual activity, perhaps because it is seen as more anti-social to introduce disease risk into what is perceived as normal sex, than to introduce risk into homosexual activity which is perceived as an abnormal, and therefore already risk-laden activity.

All the criminal prosecutions have been in relation to transmission of the HIV virus but there is no logical reason why there could not be similar prosecutions in relation to other diseases. If someone with multi-drug resistant TB were to cough or spit in a crowded room, or someone with a fever and symptoms of flu were to catch a bus, or turn up to work, or kiss a friend and pass on SARS, would these actions amount to criminal offences? Or does the stigma and discrimination which exists in relation to HIV mean that this is the only disease for which we feel sufficiently strongly about the reckless creation of risk of disease transmission to warrant prosecution? I will return to this point later.

Law's Indirect Influence on Social Norms of Behaviour

Law in the form of public health legislation and in the form of the criminal law purports to exercise direct social control. The third means of social control which might assist public health practice is by way of law's influence on public attitudes to the rightness or wrongness of behaviour.

Law is an important tool for exercising social control by indirect means. Law can serve to define relationships between members of society, and to assert what activities are permitted and what are not. If we were to subscribe to the idea of a social contract, then law is one instrument which sets out the terms of that contract.

The classic example of law's power to influence the way we behave is seat belt legislation. People now wear seat belts not because they fear prosecution but because as a society we regard the failure to wear seat belts as irresponsible. The law has changed our attitudes to car safety. The same phenomenon is now being seen in relation to legislation which prohibits smoking in public places. In countries where this has been in place for some time, such as Ireland and Australia, social attitudes to people who smoke in restaurants, or to people who smoke in public places in such a way as to invade the air space of others, have changed. Where once we may have been personally annoyed with invasive smoking, now as a society we see such smoking behaviour not just as a personal offence but as an offence against society; as irresponsible behaviour that does not accord with what we would expect of responsible members of society.

Law is a powerful dictator of social opinion, and in proscribing particular behaviours, can very quickly change public attitudes as to what is acceptable behaviour and what is not, and indeed as to what is right and what is not. Law will only operate in this way however when the law anticipates or pre-empts movement in social opinion. Law which is completely counter to cultural attitudes may have the opposite effect, mobilizing opinion into opposition to law, and making heroes of those who offend. But where law gets it right, this indirect role of law in social control might actually be the most effective mechanism at law's disposal for regulating social behaviour.

Conclusion on law as social control: law's effectiveness as a means of social control in public health We have considered three legal tools of social control: public health legislation, criminal law and law as a dictator of social attitudes. How effective is our law in social control for the benefit of the public health? Let us assume the worst, and that we are faced with human pandemic influenza in Britain. Do we have a public health legal framework which provides the powers we need to protect public health?

Firstly, because statutory duties and powers apply only to notifiable diseases, we would have to begin by giving some legal status to human pandemic influenza. Making influenza a notifiable disease would require amendment to primary legislation, which would take time and would subject the process to parliamentary debate. We could make influenza a 'disease required to be notified' under the *Public Health (Infectious Diseases) Regulations*, an easier process, and that would make the disease subject to some but not all of the provisions of the *Public Health Act*.

Once a disease is notifiable, duties of notification of disease would come into play. But one consequence of Chadwick's eagerness to keep the medical profession out of public health is that he provided that medical professionals notify disease not to a medical body but to the local authority, a body which no longer has responsibility for health. Getting the information to the place it is needed is a clumsy affair.

We would have powers of compulsory examination of persons suspected of being infected or of being exposed to influenza. This probably would not be much use in the case of influenza as anyone affected would become ill so quickly they would seek immediate medical care, and the incubation period is predicted to be short. We would have powers of compulsory isolation of a person infected with disease. The power as it is worded in our current legislation only authorizes detention to a hospital,[11] not to any other place such as detention in the home. If there were to be mass detentions, we do not have the hospital facilities to cope, and in particular we no longer have the isolation units in hospitals to enable patients to be kept isolated from other hospital patients. This lack of hospital isolation units, which resulted from the closure of isolation units after the BCG vaccine was thought to have brought tuberculosis under control, has proved a particular problem in coping with infections, ironically particularly in relation to the re-emergence of tuberculosis and multi-drug resistant tuberculosis.

What we would not have are powers of quarantine of persons who have been exposed to disease, the most useful tool in the armoury of public health officials in cases of communicable disease. We would have to amend our primary legislation to reintroduce this power. And even then, our legislation requires authorization by a JP in relation to each and every person required to remain in quarantine. There

[11] *Public Health (Control of Disease) Act 1984*, Sections 37 and 38.

are no procedures for mass quarantine outside the emergency powers which might be introduced under the *Civil Contingencies Act.*

In any event, in relation to the mechanisms we do have, there is no evidence to suggest that they work to contain disease transmission. Statutory disease reporting procedures are so clumsy that informal reporting conventions have developed parallel to compulsory notification, conventions which are more effective and which are designed with public health goals in mind. There is no longer a need for statutory surveillance mechanisms. Detention in a hospital, a measure usually disproportionate to transmission risk, has in many cases resulted in greater levels of disease transmission, both to healthcare staff and to other patients whose immune systems are likely to be lowered. Exclusion from public places might well serve some purpose, but is clumsy when the exclusion procedure must be carried out on each individual subject rather than blanket exclusions.

We would also have the possibility of prosecuting someone who exposed another to disease. Would this assist in protecting public health? The law is not a neutral instrument. The way it is framed has implications for societal beliefs and perceptions and in particular for the way society perceives the subjects of regulation. An outsider looking at our public health law would understand persons who are suffering from disease in two distinct ways: as people who are dangerous from whom we need to be protected by means of exclusion strategies, or as people who should be subject to censure and punishment. Nothing in our law would suggest that people with disease are people in need of care, treatment, sensitivity or sympathy. This in itself sends a negative public health message.

Prosecutions for reckless transmission may actually increase public health risks rather than reduce them. Criminal law does not have as its objective the protection of public health, and public health consequences do not play a part in the determination of criminality. As yet we have no research evidence to determine the public health consequences of criminalizing reckless transmission of HIV. But we can predict some possible consequences. Threat of criminal prosecution could serve as a disincentive to persons who suspect they might be HIV positive from undergoing HIV testing. Case law suggests that only persons who have been diagnosed as HIV positive will be prosecuted, so it may be safer not to know.

Prosecution may undermine trust in the confidentiality of sexual health services, such that service users are reluctant to be honest about their sexual relationships. This would inhibit use of public health tools such as contact tracing and partner notification. Persons who do engage in sexual activity which might potentially be criminal may be reluctant to advise sexual partners of the urgent need for Post-Exposure Prophylaxis, because to do so could now mean that they are admitting to a criminal offence. Criminal law intrusion into public health could put sexual partners more at risk of harm, not less. Criminalization of sexual behaviour may also serve to inhibit public health research around HIV behaviour. Researchers may be unwilling to ask questions about sexual behaviours in case the answers reveal potential criminal activity, and research subjects will be reluctant to answer.

But most importantly, such criminalization of behaviour, and the inevitable sensational media coverage, is likely to result in greater public stigma and discrimination against *all* persons who are HIV positive. Law's role as a social norm setter can work negatively as well as positively. The consequence of criminal prosecution may well have had implications for social attitudes not just in relation to the irresponsible sexual behaviour of a few HIV positive persons, but to any behaviour which is seen to create risk of transmission of the HIV virus. This can only be harmful to public health initiatives.

Law as a measure of social control could be used to public health's advantage, but it can also be used to the disadvantage of public health. The state of our present law is such that law may actually make the task of public health professionals harder. Bad law is worse than no law at all, and it may be better for law to keep out of public health altogether than to get it wrong.

I would maintain however that there is a role for law as a tool of social control, both to provide direct control through public health compulsory powers, and to provide indirect control in influencing populations to act in health-positive ways. We need to rethink what it is we need law to achieve for the benefit of public health and what law can add to existing public health strategies, and then design our new law to fulfil contemporary public health objectives.

Law as a Protector of Rights to Assist in the Provision of a Framework for Good Public Health Practice

The role of law in the protection of individual rights is another recognized function of law. Rights protection became an increasingly important component of our law over the course of the twentieth century, and particularly after the Second World War. We tend to think of law's role as a protector of rights in terms of human rights legislation, but in fact there are other, much older legal mechanisms which individuals have been able to use in pursuance of individual rights.

Law of Tort

One such mechanism is the law of tort, which enables individuals whose rights have been breached, or whose rights have been threatened, to sue for damages or an injunction. In recent years there has been a significant amount of litigation around the right to protection from public health harms, particularly in the US, where claimants have the advantage of procedural mechanisms such as the class action, and where damage awards are made by juries rather than judges.

But even within the UK we have seen some important cases where group litigation for damages for public health harms has resulted in changes to public health policy and practice.[12] The CJD litigation in 1996 in relation to the contraction of CJD from inoculation of growth hormone, resulted in changes in practice in the collection of hormones from deceased persons.[13] This was followed by litigation around new variant CJD, prompting the government to acknowledge the link between BSE in cattle and vCJD in human consumers in the establishment of a no-fault compensation scheme for sufferers of vCJD.[14] Similarly litigation against blood donation services[15] has resulted in a higher standard of care in the screening of blood for diseases such as hepatitis C, litigation against radiation services[16] has resulted in higher standards of radiation treatment for cancer, and litigation in relation to asbestos-related injuries in the workplace has resulted in significant improvement in the conditions for occupational health.[17]

But it is in the areas of obesity litigation and tobacco litigation that tort law has potential for serving as an important tool for the benefit of public health. As yet most of this litigation has been in the US,[18] but the successful cases have sent clear public health messages across the world about the acceptability of health-threatening behaviours. There have been two recipients of these messages. Firstly, the producers of products have been told that failure fully to disclose the risks associated with their products will result in costly payouts to persons who are harmed by use of the products. Secondly, consumers have been told that they no longer have to put up with misleading advertising and failure to warn of risks. Consumers of goods, like consumers of medical treatments, are entitled to make their purchase decisions on the basis of fully-informed consent, and anything less is unacceptable. There is possibly also a third recipient of the messages sent by successful tort litigation, and that is governments. Larry Gostin, the American academic who has led the revival of law as a public health tool, has pointed out that states have a moral mandate to protect the public's health.[19] The tobacco and obesity litigation has made it clear that public health laws which allow commercial enterprises to manufacture products that create risks to public health, and that

---

12 For a more detailed discussion of the role of tort in public health see R. Martin, 'Public health and the scope of potential liability in tort', *Professional Negligence*, 21/1 (2005): 39-68.

13 *N v UK Medical Research Council and Secretary of State for Health (CJD litigation)* (1996) 54 BMLR 8; [1996] Med LR 309.

14 J. Melville Williams, 'Variant Crueutzfeldt Jakob disease: setting up the vCJD trust-operation and lessons for the future', *JPIL*, 39 (2004).

15 *A v National Blood Authority* [2001] 3 All ER 289.

16 Such as *The Breast Radiation Litigation*, MedNeg Online (8 May 1998).

17 See for example *Fairchild v Glenhaven* [2003] 1 AC 32.

18 On tobacco harms see for example *Rose v Philip Morris* (29 March 2005). On obesity litigation see for example *Pelman v McDonald's Corporation* 369 F 3d 508 (25 January 2005).

19 Lawrence O. Gostin, *Public Health Law: Power, Duty, Restraint* (Berkeley: University of California Press, 2000).

allow enterprises to conceal public health risks, are flawed laws. Governments are heeding this message, and looking to their tobacco and food laws to strengthen them in the cause of improved public health.

It must be remembered that like the criminal law, tort law does not have as its objective the protection of public goods but rather is a mechanism for protecting private rights. However unlike the criminal law, tort does have the capacity to take into account wider public considerations. The criteria for determination of a tort focus on foreseeability of the damage done to the individual claimant. However refinement of tests for duty of care within the tort of negligence has allowed for public policy criteria to be taken into account in the determination of duty, such that courts could be reluctant to find a duty of care to an individual where the consequence would be a wider public harm. Nevertheless it remains the case that some tort litigation which has been brought to protect individual rights is not in the interests of the protection of public health. An example might be litigation against cervical cancer screening services for false positive cancer results. The settlement against individual claimants could well result in screening service providers withdrawing screening programmes. This would be to the detriment of women who might have had their cancer diagnosed as the result of screening.[20]

Human Rights Legislation

We cannot talk about law as a protector of rights without looking at the role of human rights legislation. The *Human Rights Act 1998* (HRA) introduced into England and Wales many of the provisions of the *European Convention of the Protection of Human Rights and Fundamental Freedoms*, enabling people whose rights have been infringed to bring actions in the domestic courts for protection of their rights. In relation to issues pertinent to public health, Article 2 (right to life), Article 3 (protection from torture and inhumane treatment), Article 5 (right to liberty) and Article 8 (right to private and family life) have been used in a range of circumstances to force public bodies to ensure that public health services respect private rights.

We have not yet had a human rights challenge to our core public health legislation, the Public Health Act. This is not because our public health legislation gives precedence to human rights. As noted earlier, our Act was framed in a spirit of utilitarianism and communitarianism, and on the assumption that private rights could be overridden whenever it was thought necessary to do so for the public good. A more likely reason why there has yet to be a human rights challenge to the exercise of powers under the Public Health Act is that the persons who are currently

---

[20] F. Stanley, 'Litigation or science?' *ALRC Reform* 69: http://www.austlii.edu.au/au/other/alrc/publications/reform/reform69/ALRCR69LITIGATIONORSCIENCE.html (accessed: 14 October 2007); E. Beerworth, 'Clinical investigations: legal implications', *Australian Prescriber*, 19 (1996): 87-8. For an example of litigation on false cancer screening results see *Penny v East Kent HA* (2000) *Lloyd's Rep Med* 41.

most usually made subject to public health powers are sufferers of tuberculosis. In the UK, as in many other states, the profile of a person with tuberculosis is likely to be someone who is homeless, poor, from a minority immigrant community, and possibly in the country illegally. Such people are rarely in a position to challenge state authority. If public health powers were to be used in cases of SARS or pandemic human influenza, then others might find themselves subject to public health powers. Such persons would have powerful ammunition for challenge under the HRA.

At this point it would be useful to look at the recent decision of the European Court of Human Rights in the case of *Enhorn v Sweden* in 2005.[21] Mr Enhorn was HIV positive, and his health behaviours such as failing to notify healthcare workers and sexual partners of his HIV status, and his lifestyle and drinking habits, caused public health concern. Eventually after public health officials had unsuccessfully tried other means of curbing his behaviour, Mr Enhorn was detained under Swedish public health legislation, legislation which is similar to our *Public Health Act* but which in fact contains a greater range of protections than does our legislation.

Mr Enhorn challenged his detention on the grounds that it breached Article 5, his right to liberty, and Article 8, his right to private and family life.[22] His challenge succeeded, and the court held that any detention under the Act was subject to two principles. The first is the principle of proportionality, such that any infringement of rights must be in proportion to the public health risk. The second is the requirement that other less restrictive means of countering the public health threat had been tried first. In other words, an exercise of powers that results in an infringement of liberty must always be a last resort. Under English public health legislation there are no powers provided for less restrictive measures. The only power available in relation to someone who presents a risk of disease transmission is isolation to a hospital, and it would be rare that a court would uphold such detention. Only in exceptional cases would such an infringement of human rights be proportional to any public health threat. It should also be noted that the procedural issues around detention under the Act, including the fact that applications for detention can be sought *ex parte*, that detention periods are not limited in the Act, and that there are no specified review or appeal processes, would almost certainly breach Article 6 of the Convention, right to a fair trial.[23]

Our public health law then does not work to protect the rights of persons suffering from disease. It is true that the common law of tort and the *Human Rights Act* enable inappropriate exercise of public health powers to be challenged,

---

21 [2005] E.C.H.R. 56529/00.

22 For a full discussion of this case see R. Martin, 'The exercise of public health powers in cases of infectious disease: human rights implications', *Medical Law Review*, 14/1 (2006): 132-43.

23 For further discussion see A. Harris and R. Martin, 'The exercise of public health powers in an era of human rights: the particular problems of tuberculosis', *Public Health*, 118/5 (2004): 313-22.

but only by those with the resources to initiate a challenge. It should not be the responsibility of individuals within the community to ensure that public health officials respect human rights, or to take action to remedy defects in our public health law. Public health legislation should itself be framed for the protection of the ill not just for the protection of the healthy, and should have as one of its objectives the provision of a framework for ethical public health practice.

Conclusion

The law that might be included in the body of what we call public health law is vast. We cannot confine public health law to our core public health legislation, although clearly the public health acts are fundamental. We must consider a broad range of laws including criminal law, tort law, environmental law, occupational health law, food law and of course laws protecting rights. Some of these laws have objectives which are consistent with the improvement of the public health. Others have entirely different objectives and their exercise in the public health domain may well be detrimental to public health.

What is lacking in our legal system, as with the legal systems of many other states, is any overarching public health legislation which makes clear public health objectives, and which makes clear the fundamental principles and values of public health endeavours in our society. Issues of legal pluralism, and the obligation to recognize differing values, will need to be addressed in the debate as to what those values are. If we want the exercise of other legal areas such as criminal law and tort law to operate consistent with public health objectives, then we need a legislative expression of those values and objectives. We are working in a legal environment where the core public health legislation no longer reflects public health practice, public health policy, public health science or community understandings of the balance between public good and private right. This has proved a significant inhibitor to the effective use of law in the pursuance of public health.

Law has enormous potential to be used for the benefit of public health. What is clear is that the importance of law as a public health tool has been underplayed and underused. While England led the way in providing legal tools for public health in the nineteenth century, it has now fallen far behind other states in the development of law which supports public health endeavour. While law is an important tool, law must also recognize and coordinate with other public health tools such as public health ethics. Law which contravenes societal conceptions of ethics and human rights will not change public health behaviours, but rather will entrench dangerous public health behaviours.

Many states are in the process of amending their public health laws. New Zealand and Western Australia for example, both of which have laws based on the *1875 English Public Health Act*, have prepared consultation papers which propose entirely new conceptions of public health law in accordance with contemporary science, values, ethics and rights. There is much to be done in this jurisdiction to make full use of law as a public health tool. I would urge that it should be done, and done soon, before we find ourselves faced with a new and overwhelming public health challenge.

Chapter 3
Luck, Risk and Prevention

Katherine King
London School of Economics, UK and New York University, USA

Preventing disadvantage would certainly seem to be a central goal of egalitarian social policy. Nowhere is this preference for prevention more vividly illustrated than in the sphere of health, where prevention is pursed primarily through public health policy, and compensation, through the acute treatment of illness by physicians and other healthcare workers. These preventive interventions are both more efficient and thorough than acute treatment. Indeed, the dramatic improvements in both health and lifespan witnessed over the last century are due not so much to technological advancements in the acute treatment of illness, but to improvements in our ability to prevent disease through immunizations, improved nutrition and sanitation and other mechanisms of public health policy.[1] These policies are also a more thorough response to disease. Even when treatment is fully effective, it cannot remove the pain and suffering caused by illness.

The strong pull of prevention does not mean that it will always be the appropriate response. Often harm and disadvantage result from our own choices. Preventing those hardships would entail restricting choice. To the extent that such choice is valued, prevention could be a problematic response. Similarly, in blocking outcomes, prevention can be insulting and paternalistic, particularly in cases where there is disagreement about whether the condition is in fact a disadvantage.

These complexities aside, prevention would seem to be an important part of egalitarian social policy, and over the course of this paper, I will explore its role. In particular, I will focus on the luck-egalitarian approach to distributive justice. Because it is structured as a response to uncertainty, it would seem to invite a preventive orientation. However, I will argue that while opening the door to preventive responses, luck-egalitarianism ultimately fails to realize this potential because of an attenuated understanding of uncertainty. I will then move on to offer a refined account that can potentially recognize the place of prevention in distributive justice.

---

1 US Department of Health and Human Services, Office of Disease Control and Prevention, *For a Healthy Nation: Returns on Investment in Public Health* (Washington, DC: US Department of Health and Human Services, 1995).

Preliminary Distinctions

Fundamentally, the distinction between prevention and compensation is temporal. Compensation responds to existing disadvantage and prevention to its possibility. A canonical example of compensation would be giving wheelchairs to individuals with decreased mobility. In this instance, as in many cases of compensation, the good is distributed in response to an existent hardship precisely to those individuals in need. In contrast immunizations are a paradigmatic example of prevention, as when immunized, the individual is not experiencing any disadvantage. Nevertheless, they are immunized with the hope of staving off disease.

In practice, the distinction between compensation and prevention is not always so stark. Often, the same intervention is both preventive and compensatory. Trivially, this will always be the case; if a hungry man is given food, his current hunger is satiated, but so too is the hunger that he would have had in an hour. Here, the connection is trivial because the compensation is preventive only in that it blocks the continuance of the same disadvantage in the same individual, and if it did not accomplish this feat, we would hardly have considered the intervention compensatory in the first place. In other cases, however, the interaction is much more complex. In particular, compensation can prevent the same or different disadvantages for the same or different individuals.

For example, nutrition programmes for infants exemplify compensatory policies that are compensatory and preventive for different disadvantages in the same person. These programmes directly respond to the existent disadvantage of insufficient food in the infants, and in this sense are compensatory. However, in so doing, they also prevent a host of health and developmental problems that the children could potentially suffer as a result of their poor nutrition in infancy, such as lowered IQ. Alternatively, risk-exposure can itself be understood as a disadvantage. For instance, it can cause fear and anxiety that lead to negative behavioural changes. These consequences of risk are existent disadvantages caused by the possibility of future, but distinct disadvantage. Consequently, to the extent that any preventive policy also assuages these existing cognitive and behavioral stresses it can be understood in compensatory terms as well.

In other policies, the preventive and compensatory effects of a policy are not necessarily experienced by the same people. Consider, for example, a regulation requiring all public buildings to be accessible by wheelchairs. In the first instance, this policy is compensatory, responding to the existing difficulty that those in wheelchairs face accessing buildings. However, now that the buildings are wheelchair accessible, others who find themselves in wheelchairs in the future will not suffer the same access difficulties that they would have before the regulation was passed, and in this sense, the policy is preventive for the same disability in other people. In this case, the disadvantage being compensated and prevented is the same, however, this need not always be the case. In responding to the existing disadvantage in educational opportunities experienced by African-Americans, the desegregation of American schools challenged the dominant prejudices against the

African-American population, contributing to greater social respect and equality for group as a whole. As these examples illustrate, compensatory policies that have these more general preventive effects will most often take the form of what Wolff has referred to as 'status enhancement', adjusting social and material structures so that a particular characteristic is no longer experienced as a disadvantage.[2]

Luck, Choice and Prevention

Given the general orientation towards equality-of-opportunity approaches in contemporary distributive justice, one appealing possibility is that prevention can be addressed through an opportunity-based framework. The plausibility of this suggestion is further strengthened by the intuitive link between the two. Both opportunity and prevention imply a capacity to control or constrain future uncertainty. However, the idea of opportunity is notoriously vague. In order to see whether this similarity can be exploited to integrate prevention into distributive justice, we need to focus more narrowly, and the target I will focus on is opportunity within luck-egalitarianism.

The intuitive core of luck-egalitarianism is a belief that the course of an individual's life ought to be determined by choice, whereas the impact of chance ought to be mitigated. On this reading, opportunity is understood as a matter of individual choice; to the extent that individuals make choices determining their future, they have opportunity. Conversely, to the extent that factors other than their choices shape their lives, they lack opportunity. In general, theorists have referred to the lack of opportunity as 'luck'. Given this distinction between choice and luck, equality is conceptualized as ensuring that the scope of choice in determining our lives is equal, whereas the impact of luck is mitigated as far as possible.[3] [4] [5]

The luck-egalitarian concern with chance and uncertainty preserves the intuitive connection between opportunity and prevention noted above. However, over the course of the following section, I will argue that the characterization of uncertainty in terms of luck is too attenuated to allow for preventive intervention. To present these arguments, I will focus specifically on Ronald Dworkin's account. His suggestions are particularly interesting to consider as his responses to luck—choice and insurance—are similar to contemporary arguments being made about prevention in the context of health.

Dworkin offers two responses to uncertainty, which map onto a distinction in the kinds of luck we face. On the one hand, there is 'option-luck', which

---

[2] J. Wolff, 'Disability Among Equals': http://www.homepages.ucl.ac.uk/~uctyjow/DAE.doc (accessed 24/10/06).

[3] R. Dworkin, *Sovereign Virtue* (Cambridge: Harvard University Press, 2000).

[4] G.A. Cohen, 'On the Currency of Egalitarian Justice', *Ethics*, 99 (1999): 906-44.

[5] R. Arneson, 'Equality and Equal Opportunity for Welfare', *Philosophical Studies*, 56 (1989): 77-93.

encompasses all uncertainty that is introduced into our lives through choice, such as freely and deliberately chosen gambles and bets that should have been anticipated and could have been declined.[6] While we do not control the outcomes of option-luck, because it is introduced through individual choice, at one point we did have control. In contrast to option-luck is 'brute-luck', which is characterized negatively as all uncertainty that did not result from deliberate and calculated gambles. Being struck by a meteorite or being born with Huntington's disease are both canonical examples of bad brute-luck. Admittedly, option- and brute-luck are extremes on a spectrum, with most instances of luck falling in between.[7]

The presence of option-luck does not raise much concern for the luck-egalitarian. It is in our life because of choice. As such, it reflects preferences, which are dimensions of a life that the individual should and usually does take responsibility for. Accordingly, differences emanating from them do not raise concerns of justice. Brute-luck however, is more of a challenge because it does not reflect the individual's choices, but rather mere chance, and it seems inherently unjust that one should be disadvantaged due to no fault of her own.

In response to this injustice, Dworkin argues that its impact needs to be mitigated. It can be mitigated, or so he argues, through insurance. Insurance provides a link between option- and brute-luck by hedging the impact of bad brute-luck through a calculated choice, *ex ante*. In deciding to purchase insurance, the individual evaluates the significance of the particular bad brute-luck in her life. She then weighs the cost of suffering the harm and the likelihood of it coming to pass against the cost of insurance and the potential compensation. In buying insurance, brute-luck is transformed into option-luck because now the individual has made a choice about the consequences of possible bad luck in her life.

Prima facie, insurance looks preventive. It is a decision made *ex ante* in response to an uncertain future that introduces a degree of control. Ultimately however, this potential is not realized as the kind of control insurance introduces does not allow for prevention, but only *ex ante* agreement about the *ex post* compensatory response that should take place if the undesirable event comes to pass. The control it offers is not control over the undesirable event, but rather control over its consequences. In contrast, prevention is explicitly concerned with controlling the undesirable event itself. Unemployment insurance does not prevent unemployment but only its financial consequences; auto insurance does not prevent car accidents, but rather mitigates their financial impact.

Could it be that we were looking in the wrong place for Dworkin's preventive strategies and that prevention is addressed in the context of option-luck? If option-luck is Dworkin's response to prevention, then prevention is primarily a question of individual choice. To a certain extent this seems reasonable. There are many forms of disadvantage that are preventable through individual choice. While there

6 Dworkin, *Sovereign Virtue*.

7 Ibid., p. 73.

are many disadvantages choice cannot prevent, option-luck looks like it is at least part of a solution.

If, however, option-luck is the way Dworkin conceptualizes prevention, we are again left empty-handed. Option-luck is a matter of individual choice. It is a choice made in the light of individual preferences and understanding of the good. These personal judgments and their consequences are simply not a matter of justice but belong in the sphere of the personal, just like choices regarding religion and one's family. But, if prevention is a means for achieving distributive equality, there must be the possibility of influencing its distribution in the population through government intervention, and it is precisely this interference that is closed off in the case of option-luck. Moreover, the distinction between option- and brute-luck was introduced precisely to recognize individual responsibility for preferences. Accordingly, it is not only paternalistic but also counter to the motivation of option-luck to see it as the subject of further redistribution.

Consequently, we are left with a fairly negative conclusion about Dworkin's capacity to address prevention. On the one hand, his response to brute-luck, e.g. insurance, is not a form of prevention but an *ex ante* way of settling on *ex post* levels of compensation in response to disadvantage that has already materialized. As such, there is no effort to mitigate or otherwise control its likelihood, as would be required of prevention. In contrast, risks associated with option-luck can be influenced and therefore hold out the possibility of prevention. However, to the extent that distributive justice is concerned with prevention, this door too is closed because these choices are a matter of individual responsibility so not the concern of egalitarian redistribution.

The inability to address preventive concerns within luck-egalitarianism is surprising. The account was motivated precisely to mitigate bad luck. This goal would seem to invite two strategies: lessen the consequences of bad luck or eradicate it ensuring that the luck was never experienced in the first place. Yet while there are these two possibilities, Dworkin's account focuses entirely on the first, compensatory strategy, disregarding the later, preventive approach. In the context of his argument Dworkin might be thought to address this concern through his assumption that in the canonical moment of equality in the auction, all participants face the *same antecedent risks* to their wellbeing, making all prevention simply a matter of choice in this context.[8] However, given his concern with responding to luck, and addressing unequal luck, this idealization seems particularly unjustified and problematic.

Risks, Causes and Groups

While ultimately Dworkin's argument does not allow for preventive responses, the shortcomings his frameworks encounter do provide a roadmap for how to move

[8] Ibid., p. 77.

forward. In particular, we found that the categories of brute- and option-luck were too impoverished to invite a concern with prevention. The uncertainty under them was either brute and beyond our control, or the result of choice and hence wholly within our control. In order to recognize prevention, this framework would have to be enhanced. Second, I noted that this exclusive orientation towards compensatory responses was facilitated in the context of his argument because its need was simply assumed away in the canonical moment of equality. This later difficulty is readily addressed by giving up the assumption of equal antecedent risk. However, the former challenge of enriching the distinction between brute- and option-luck requires more consideration.

In thinking about how to enhance this distinction, consider two *prima facie* targets for prevention. First, take the case of an individual who develops an E. coli infection after eating bad spinach. It is very likely that this bad luck could not have been anticipated or avoided by the individual, and so would be classified as brute-luck. Yet while this disease was seemingly random, and hence not preventable from the individual's perspective, it may very well have been preventable, for example through better food inspection or through tighter regulations on the growing of spinach. Next, consider a case of option-luck, such as the choice to start smoking. On the above account, a choice such as this would be a classic example of option-luck, and accordingly, taken to be immune from government intervention. But certainly such immunity is only a half-truth as smoking is widely believed to be the number one preventable cause of disease in America and Europe. Moreover, as aggressive anti-smoking policies demonstrate, there are many actions governments can take to prevent that choice, such as counteracting tobacco advertising with graphic health warnings on cigarette packages and restricting smoking in public places.

These examples highlight that in cases of both *prima facie* option- and brute-luck, prevention is possible. In recognizing this possibility, the earlier framework is enriched, incorporating factors beyond individual choice and mere randomness. In the case of E. coli, for example, prevention is possible when the disease is no longer seen as simply bad luck, but is understood as the predictable result of an identified causal agent that could become the target of preventive interventions. Again with smoking, the possibility for prevention emerged when we ceased to see the choice as simply the outcome of internal deliberative processes and recognized influences on that choice beyond individual preferences, such as exposure to tobacco advertising, and the social acceptability of smoking. In pursuing prevention, it is these factors, and not the individual's choice *per se*, that become the targets of intervention.

To recognize these factors, and integrate an explicit concern with prevention, I suggest that we first have to move away from the concept of 'luck'. Luck has long been used in moral theory as a catch-all for all myriad events in our lives that are unexpected, and as a catch-all it has rarely been rigorously characterized. Even in luck-egalitarianism where luck is a central concept, it is only characterized negatively, defined as whatever the individual is not responsible for.[9] What is determining the outcome is left unspecified. This oversight is unfortunate because there are many causes of disadvantage beyond individual choices that are relevant to distributive justice.[10] [11] Simply lumping them together as the result of luck obscures this complexity and its relevance to moral theory. Consequently, to the extent that we are concerned with the cause of a disadvantage, as I have suggested we ought to be in pursing prevention, 'luck' is a particularly inopportune concept.

A more appropriate concept to be working with would be *risk*. Like luck, risk refers to uncertainty about the future. However, risk is more structured, and structured in ways that facilitate decisions about prevention. In particular, risk-statements identify factors that either predict or cause the disadvantage in question, and either implicitly or explicitly indicate our uncertainty about the postulated connection. Moreover, risk is also a feature of groups as opposed to individuals, which as I will argue, is a central feature of preventive responses.

As argued above, preventive responses require that we identify targets of intervention. Unlike statements about luck, statements about risk facilitate this inference by connecting risk factors with outcomes. In many cases, this inference is causal. However, risk factors need not causally contribute to the disadvantage to aid in preventive interventions. Rather, by flagging at-risk populations, they can simply direct resources to that group. Causal inferences in risk-analysis raise a number of concerns, and while there are genuine difficulties here, the problems are often overstated. The causal inferences involved in risk analyses are not simply the result of statistical correlation, but rather reflect significant 'extra-statistical' information ranging from the consistency, sensitivity and temporality of the association to knowledge about the causal structure of the event gleaned through experimentation and experience.

From the perspective of the egalitarian, a more serious problem presented by causal inferences in risk-analysis is determining which risk factors ought to be identified and targeted. When we ask the question of why an individual developed lung cancer after a lifetime of smoking, there are many ways to describe them. These possibilities fall into three broad categories: (1) *personal*, such as the individual's preferences and self-esteem/self-image; (2) *social*, such as who the individual's friends are, and social norms about smoking; and (3) *environmental*, such as the accessibility of tobacco and the prevalence of tobacco advertising and promotion in the community, or the legal and regulatory structure surrounding tobacco. These categories are not mutually exclusive and often a single risk factor can be understood as falling into many categories simultaneously. For example,

9 S.L. Hurley, *Justice, Luck, and Knowledge* (Cambridge: Harvard University Press, 2003).

10 A. Phillips, 'Defending Equality of Outcome', *Journal of Political Philosophy*, 12/1 (2004): 1-19.

11 I.M. Young, 'Equality of Whom? Social Groups and Judgments of Injustice', *The Journal of Political Philosophy*, 9 (2001): 1-18.

low self-esteem could be read as both a personal factor and a social factor. How we choose to describe them will be very important as each account will carry with it distinct implications about the nature of intervention pursued.

A further advantage in working with the concept of risk is that it makes explicit the extent and nature of uncertainty associated with making preventive decisions. This uncertainty may be of two sorts: there may be uncertainty about the existence of a causal relation between the risk factor and outcome, and the relationship between the risk factor and outcome may be genuine but probabilistic. These considerations are central to decisions about preventive interventions. All things equal, the less likely the outcome, the less likely we are to feel that preventive interventions are called for.

A final advantage of a risk-based perspective is that it makes explicit the kind of group-orientation, which, I would argue, is crucial to prevention. This group orientation can factor into preventive interventions in at least two key ways. First, a group-orientation is central to the predictive inferences that guide prevention. Second, many of the causes targeted by prevention are more appropriately understood as operating at the level of groups, as opposed to individuals.

Any preventive intervention is grounded on an inference predicting who is likely to experience the relevant disadvantage. This capacity for prediction can only be realized by adopting a group-perspective. When we consider individuals one at a time, we have no ability to predict who will suffer a disadvantage and who will not. It is only by considering those individuals as members of a group, sharing a particular risk factor that we can make predictions. For example, while we can say that as a smoker, Tom has a 50 per cent chance of developing lung cancer; it is only by considering Tom as a member of a larger group, namely smokers, that we are able to make this prediction. In this context, groups, or risk-groups, are defined by identifying those populations that demonstrate a similar propensity to the disadvantage of interest *because of* the presence of a common influence, i.e. risk factor. Accordingly, the groups can be identified by any characteristic that is reasonably identified as a risk factor.

Importantly, because these predictions are at the group-level, prevention will also have an over-corrective nature, directing us to those groups, not individuals, in need of preventive interventions. That is, all individuals in the identified group will be considered disadvantaged (i.e. recipients of the preventive intervention) even if they do not currently suffer any hardship because of the risk, and recognizing that even without the intervention, would never have experienced the projected hardship. Rather, their categorization as disadvantaged and their priority in redistribution is established from their membership in that high-risk group.

There are many different ways that a group of individuals can face the same risk, and we would not consider all of them to be cases of group-luck. In a lottery, for example, many individuals face the same risk simultaneously, yet a lottery is the epitome of individual, option-luck. However, the risk in a lottery is only common because each individual made a separate, isolated decision to enter into that risk. For that reason, it is the individual's choice and not her membership of any particular group that determines her risk exposure. Similarly, in cases of pure-individualized brute-luck, such as getting hit by a meteorite, there is no insight gained by adopting a group perspective, except perhaps learning that the event is random. However, when we turn to cases of genuine group-luck, to the extent that an individual chooses that group membership, the choice was not an isolated gamble to assume a risk, and in many cases such as membership in a sociodemographic, the individual does not even have this choice to enter into the group. Accordingly the ensuing risks are misdescribed as instances of option-luck.

In understanding them as risks, however, we can walk a middle ground between these two extremes, recognizing these influences as risk, operating within a group that constrain but do not necessarily determine the outcome. Consider again the choice to start smoking. There are a number of clearly identified risk factors that make this choice more likely. An individual is more likely to start smoking if her friends or parents smoke, if cigarette advertising targets her sociodemographic, or if she lives in a society with permissive norms and laws about smoking. What is notable about all of these causes is that they impact individuals in virtue of their membership in a particular group. That is, membership is itself a factor in their risk exposure. It is sociodemographics that are targeted by advertising, and if a peer-group glamorizes smoking, the entire group faces the risk in virtue of their membership in that group. That is, once a member of the group, the individual will often be exposed to risks over which they have no direct control. In noting these group-level influences, I do not mean to deny the presence of individual choice or suggest that the presence of such group-level influences somehow absolves the individual of responsibility. The individual still faces choices. In the case of smoking, the individual chose to start smoking; she chooses not to quit, and she chooses to spend her money on cigarettes. Yet while she has choices, those choices, and her preferences in relation to those choices are being structured by her group membership. Group membership might, for example, present the individual with choices, option-luck that she might not have faced if she had been in a different group. Moreover, it might increase the costs of making certain choices. For example, if none of her friends smoke, she might never be presented with the choice to start herself, or alternatively, if all of her friends smoke, the choice not to smoke might have additional costs, such as social exclusion, costs that an individual with different friends might not have to bear.

One possible response is to argue that these structures ought to be considered instances of brute-luck. In addition to the concerns about the brute-luck expressed earlier, however such a response is too severe. The classification of these choices as brute-luck implies that the individual bears no responsibility for her choices. Not only does such a move alienate the individual, making her a victim of her circumstance, but it also does not seem quite right. These group-factors do not remove individual choice, but rather influence it. Instead of viewing the influences as removing individual choice and responsibility, the risk perspective encourages us to recognize an intermediate position in which risks do not remove individual responsibility, so much as mitigate it.

It is this middle ground, between luck and choice, and between individual and the group responsibility that is crucial to recognizing the possibility of prevention and integrating it into an egalitarian response to disadvantage. While existing arguments in the luck-egalitarian literature have difficulty accommodating this complexity, I have argued that a shift towards risk, as opposed to luck, both creates this space and structures preventive responses by identifying contributing factors and groups who may be in need of prevention, as well as flagging our own uncertainty about the relationship.

Chapter 4
The Duty to Promote Social Capital

Patricia Illingworth
Northeastern University, Boston, USA

In November 2002, the Chinese government suppressed information about the outbreak of a respiratory disease in Guangdong Province. Despite the efforts of the Chinese government to keep information secret, the information leaked through various Internet sources. On 11 February 2003, after being approached by the World Health Organization[1], China disclosed that there was, indeed, an outbreak of SARS in Guangdong Province that had resulted in about 300 cases and five deaths. Between February and April 2003, although the Chinese Government acknowledged the outbreak of SARS, they undertook to cover up the extent of it. Among other things, they prohibited state-controlled media from reporting on the outbreak.

More recently, concerned with the outbreak of avian flu, some corporations attempted to hoard Tamiflu, the primary medication thought to be effective in treating the flu. Pharmaceutical companies are loathe to forfeit their patents on essential medicines for fear of compromising their profit margin; globally, they have been slow to undertake the challenge of meeting the need to create drugs for neglected diseases that afflict millions of the sick and poor. And of course, all of us have collectively failed to adequately respond to world poverty.

Today, philosophers, and in particular those working in applied ethics and social and political philosophy can often achieve the greatest impact on social problems by working with people from other disciplines, and government and non-government organizations. As we consider what obligations the state has to the community, individuals to each other, and one nation to the other, it may be worthwhile to explore nontraditional conceptual tools. In this paper, I argue that the concept of social capital, though traditionally a sociological, economic and, more recently, public health concept, should also be understood as an ethical one, one that has promising implications for applied ethics, health care ethics, and global justice. The concept of social capital has been strongly endorsed by the World Bank, and by many governments worldwide—Australia, Ireland, and Canada, to name a few. According to a recent World Bank document, 'social capital is a concept that has significant implications for enhancing the quality,

---

[1] WHO (World Health Organization), *International Nurse Mobility: Trends and Implications* (Geneva: WHO, 2003). Available at: http://whqlibdoc.who.int/hq/2003/WHO_EIP_OSD_2003.3.pdf (accessed 13 June 2006).

effectiveness and sustainability of World Bank operations, particularly those that are based on community action.'[2] The concept of social capital, like the concept of liberty, is valuable because of what it enables. Liberty gives individuals the opportunity to satisfy their conceptions of the good; social capital, and the social trust that accompanies it, gives them the wherewithal to work collaboratively with others, in order to enjoy the fruits that accompany cooperation with people.

In what follows, I will first define the concept of social capital, drawing on the work of an interdisciplinary group of scholars. This definition, though admittedly imprecise, provides us with a good understanding of the morally relevant aspects of the concept of social capital. Second, I will explain in what way social capital qualifies as a moral concept. Third, I discuss the possibility of building global social capital, and the potential difficulties with that enterprise.

Social Capital

The concept of social capital has a long and distinguished history, beginning in the early twentieth century, when education reformers used it to encourage participation in schools. According to J. Coleman,

> Social capital is defined by its function. It is not a single entity, but a variety of different entities claiming two characteristics in common: they all consist of some aspect of social structure, and they facilitate certain actions of individuals who are within the structure. Like other forms of capital, social capital is productive, making possible the achievement of certain ends that would not be attainable in its absence.[3]

More recently, Francis Fukuyama and Robert Putnam have popularized the concept of social capital.[4] Lisa Berkman and Ichiro Kawachi have noted three generalizations common to various definitions of social capital. First, social capital is social—that is, it is 'a feature of the collective (neighbourhood, community,

2 World Bank, *Overview: Social Capital* (Washington: World Bank Group, 2006). Available at: http://web.worldbank.org/WBSITE/EXTERNAL/TOPICS/EXTSOCIALDEVELOPMENT/EXTTSOCIALCAPITAL/0,,contentMDK:20642703~menuPK:401023~pagePK:148956~piPK:216618~theSitePK:401015,00.html (accessed 19 June 2006).

3 J.S. Coleman, *Foundations of Social Theory* (Cambridge, MA: Belknap Press of Harvard University Press, 1994).

4 F. Fukuyama, *Trust: The Social Virtues and the Creation of Prosperity* (New York: Free Press, 1996).

society) to which the individual belongs'.[5] Second, they have noted that it is a public good. Moreover, it should be viewed as a 'byproduct of social relationships'.[6]

Social capital creates the possibility of productive, cooperative activity. According to Putnam, social capital consists of the 'networks, norms, and social trust that facilitate coordination and cooperation for mutual benefit'. For Putnam, important indicators of social capital are levels of trust, perceived reciprocity and the extent of membership in civic associations. Social capital can be viewed as one of the benefits that 'flow from the trust, reciprocity, information, and cooperation associated with social networks. Social capital creates value for the people who are connected and at least sometimes for bystanders'.[7]

Three important indicators of social capital are: (1) norms, values and attitudes, (2) networks and (3) consequences.[8] Trust is a crucial attitude for the creation of social capital. It has the potential to transform self-interested and self-seeking actors into collaborators and cooperators. Because of this, the extent of trust in a relationship is often a good measure of the degree of social capital present. Trust facilitates generalized reciprocity. In turn, generalized reciprocity takes interpersonal relations outside of a tit-for-tat exchange in which people require an immediate return on their 'gifts'. When people are part of a community in which generalized reciprocity governs their interactions, they know that they will be a beneficiary at some later time, and perhaps from another person altogether. Without trust, generalized reciprocity would be impossible, and without generalized reciprocity, there would be little or no social capital. The willingness of people to undertake a burden hinges on trusting that they will be a beneficiary of similar kindness in the future.

Networks can be a very tangible form of social capital, as in the case of an extensive list of personal and professional contacts. People with wide networks can more effectively advance themselves professionally and socially. Social networks are important for individual health and wellbeing. Because networks convey the message that strangers can be 'relied on' for kindness, they also create social capital for the community.[9] Social capital is thought to have a number of positive consequences, including 'mutual support, cooperation, trust and institutional effectiveness'.[10] It has been found to be important for preventing delinquency, improving education and community life, and in criminology.[11]

---

5 L.F. Berkman and I. Kawachi, *Social Epidemiology* (New York: Oxford University Press, 2000).

6 Ibid.

7 R.D. Putnam, *Bowling Alone: The Collapse and Revival of American Community* (New York: Simon & Schuster, 2001).

8 K. Newton, 'Social Capital and Democracy', *American Behavioral Scientist*, 40 (1997): 575-86.

9 Putnam, *Bowling Alone*.

10 Ibid., p. 22.

11 Berkman and Kawachi, *Social Epidemiology*, p. 174; P. Illingworth, *Trusting Medicine* (New York: Routledge, 2005), p. 93.

Other scholars, such as Robison and Flora, have identified a social capital paradigm that has two main components.[12] These authors describe social capital as 'sympathy toward another person or group that may produce a potential benefit, advantage, and preferential treatment for another person or groups beyond that expected in an exchange relationship', and 'socio-emotional goods that are expressed emotions between persons that validate or provide information that increases self-awareness or self-regard',[13]

Additionally, two different *types* of social capital have been identified by Putnam: 'bonding' and 'bridging'. Bonding social capital reinforces the *inward* perspective of a group, and it can be found in homogenous groups, such as fraternal organizations.[14] Unlike bridging social capital, bonding social capital can breed exclusivity among relatively insular groups. Nonetheless, it provides support for members of the group. Historically, it has been facilitated by the 'thick trust' of face-to-face interactions within primary relations.[15]

Bridging social capital, facilitated by 'thin trust', is the glue that links people within different groups to each other. Thin trust, unlike thick trust, fosters a willingness to trust people outside of our immediate circle.[16] Bridging social capital is valuable precisely because it builds bridges between groups and enhances the willingness of people 'to give most [people]—even those whom they do not know from direct experience—the benefit of the doubt'.[17] Because bridging social capital promotes tolerance and empathy, it is particularly important in a society as diverse as ours and in the global scheme.[18]

Trust and social capital go hand in hand. According to Fukuyama, social capital is 'a capability that arises from the prevalence of trust in society'.[19] It is facilitated by the shared norms permitting 'regular and honest cooperative behaviour'.[20] Moreover, trust facilitates generalized reciprocity, which is the touchstone of social capital. Social capital should be understood as the product of cooperation among people, and cooperation depends on the existence of trust.

Trust is also a social good. According to Bok, 'trust is a social good to be protected just as much as the air we breathe or the water we drink. When it is damaged, the community as a whole suffers and when it is destroyed, societies

---

12 L.J. Robison and J.L. Flora, 'The Social Capital Paradigm: Bridging Across Disciplines', *American Journal of Agricultural Economics*, 85 (2003): 1208-10.

13 Ibid., p. 1209.

14 Putnam, *Bowling Alone*.

15 Newton, 'Social Capital and Democracy', pp. 575-86.

16 Putnam, *Bowling Alone*, p. 136.

17 Ibid.

18 P. Illingworth, *Trusting Medicine: The Moral Costs of Managed Care* (London: Routledge, 2005), pp. 93-4.

19 Fukuyama, *Trust*.

20 Ibid.

falter and collapse'.[21] A similar theme appears in much of the literature on social capital. Social capital and trust are genuine public goods insofar as social relations create them indirectly, and the benefits from them cannot be restricted only to those who have contributed to their cultivation. In the case of private goods such as a piece of chocolate, a transfer of the good can be restricted to the purchaser. It is excludable (we are able to exclude others from having it) and rivalrous. Public goods are non-excludable and non-rivalrous. In the classic case of a traffic light, for example, the benefit of the light cannot be restricted to just the person who is using it (non-rivalrous) and is non-excludable because it would be extraordinarily expensive to restrict usage to one person or group. Social capital is similar. It is non-rivalrous in the sense that one person's use of social capital (networks, norms, social trust) does not entail that others cannot use it and, though bonding social capital can become somewhat insular, that insularity would seem not to be endemic to social capital. It would take considerable effort to exclude people from accessing the available social capital.[22] Free riders, individuals, and institutions, who, for example, have not contributed to the 'trust fund', can often draw on its wealth. The relationship between trust and social capital is complex. Trust is a component or mark of social capital, but is also independent of it.

The World Bank has added to this understanding of social capital the idea that trust and solidarity go hand in hand, and both enhance social cohesion and collective action. They also add social cohesion and inclusion because, in their words, this 'mitigates the risk of conflict and promotes equitable access to development by enhancing participation of the marginalized'.[23] Finally, they add, 'information and communication break down negative social capital and also enable positive social capital by improving access to information'.[24] Although the concept of social capital is imprecise, and frustrating especially for philosophers because of that imprecision, it appears to refer to a cluster of concepts that are helpful in understanding the contribution of social interaction to a productive life and community welfare that may otherwise not be acknowledged. We cannot have social capital in a world populated by selfish and self- interested people. Moral philosophers and applied ethicists need to join the ongoing conversation about social capital and embrace the concept, because doing so increases the likelihood that people will treat their fellow human beings with more concern. Thus, I will argue that ethics, social and political philosophy, and the law are good homes for social capital.

---

[21] S. Bok, *Lying* (London: Quartet Books Limited, 1978).

[22] Inge Kaul, Isabelle Grunberg and Marc A. Stern (eds), *Global Public Goods* (New York: Oxford University Press, 1999).

[23] World Bank, *Social Capital.*

[24] Ibid.

Social Capital as an Ethical Concept

Together, ethics, the law and policy govern interactions among people. Moral philosophy and applied ethics are concerned with the ethical quality of these interactions. To say that a concept or principle is ethical is to say, at the very least, that it refers to something which is generally regarded as good, that overall, it is worthy of pursuit, and that it would be better to have it than not to have it. This is not to say that it is *the* most important value, because, like other ethical principles and concepts, there will be times when social capital conflicts with other values—all morally worthwhile pursuits—and we will need to make choices in order to balance these. Most obviously, social capital may conflict with negative liberty, though this conflict is not a logical or analytical one.

Social capital is like the concept of liberty: it is an enabler concept, valuable for what it produces. Liberty, as we know from Mill's discussion in *On Liberty*, is important because among other things, people know themselves best, and therefore should be given the latitude to choose their own life plans.[25] Mill seemed to believe that if we ultimately want to maximize happiness, it is best to give people freedom. Here liberty is not valuable for its own sake but for what it can produce. Similarly, people who are flush with social capital are in a better position to secure the benefits that accompany social trust, cohesiveness, and solidarity.

Although there is no consensus about what counts as an ethical concept, there are a number of characteristics typically associated with them. First, ethical concepts usually concern conduct towards others.[26] Since social capital is a product of the relationships between and among people, it certainly involves conduct towards others. Other regarding conduct is also reflected in generalized reciprocity, which, after all, advocates the idea that people ought to give to others even when they cannot anticipate in kind immediate, and direct reciprocation.

Second, ethical concepts are universal: if a concept, principle, or value is an ethical one, then what it dictates will be true for everyone.[27] Universalization can be understood in a number of ways. Peter Singer has provided a helpful discussion in his book, *Practical Ethics*. Although it is not clear how one would universalize social capital, the concept of liberty can again be instructive. Like liberty, social capital seems to be important for everyone. Though people possess different amounts of social capital (as they do liberty), and different psychological capacities to take advantage of it, access to social capital seems to be universally valuable. Moreover, the notion of generalized reciprocity which is embedded within the concept of social capital is similar to the golden rule. We can call it the Rule of Generalized Reciprocity: 'give even when you cannot anticipate reciprocity'.

Third, ethical statements are prescriptive. That is, if a concept is an ethical one, then to say that it is ethical is also to say something like 'it is good', or 'do x'.

---

25 J.S. Mill, *On Liberty* (1859) (New York: Penguin Books, 1975).

26 P. Singer, *Practical Ethics* (Cambridge, UK: Cambridge University Press, 1993).

27 Ibid.

Social capital also satisfies this condition. Although social capital may have a dark side (excluding others in the case of bonding social capital), overall, it is a good thing, and it is regarded as such. Social capital is productive of goods that we value. Ethical statements are also normative. They are not descriptive statements, but state what ought to be the case. Insofar as social capital is used to promote good ends (and not, for example, to promote the racists goals of the Ku Klux Klan), it is implied that it ought to be pursued.

Thus far, I have looked at the formal qualities characteristic of the ethical. The concept of social capital also has substantive ethical qualities. Social capital is communitarian or social. It is *of* the people, and *for* the people. Social capital cannot be produced by one person; it is not the stuff of rugged individualism, but rather, the stuff of community relations, in which people act for each other and in solidarity. A society with a strong commitment to negative liberty may find it difficult, though not impossible, to cultivate social capital. Social capital needs to be nurtured at the very least by putting people together. Although face-to-face interactions are important for the cultivation of social capital, a thoughtful approach may help to identify other methods that may be more appropriate to a global world, such as widespread use of the Internet.

Social capital is also an ethical concept insofar as it carries with it a particular vision of responsibility. Consider again a comparison with the concept of liberty. Arguably, the concept of individual liberty implies that *individuals* are responsible for their actions. Social capital seems to suggest that many outcomes, which we typically associate with individual action, may more accurately be understood as the result of collaborations or cooperative actions. The legal concept of 'but for' causation may artificially focus attention on the actions of one person or one action, often neglecting the input of the collective. The concept of social capital might be better complemented by a different notion of causation, one that incorporates the indirect causation that Elizabeth Ashford has so carefully analyzed.[28] For example, the good health that some people experience may not be the result of individual actions but more accurately the social networks available to them. Similarly, the longer life spans of women may be the result of their more extensive access to social networks. A deep understanding of the presence of social capital in a community may lift outcomes out of the moral paradigm of individual responsibility and place them in the paradigm of collaboration or collective responsibility.

Social capital also implicates another moral concept, that of justice. Justice is concerned with the distribution of burdens and benefits in society. Social capital is both a benefit to be distributed and a mechanism for distributing prized benefits. As Putnam points out, those with a more extensive Rolodex enjoy greater social capital and the benefits it engenders.[29] Because of the substantial gains associated

---

[28] E. Ashford, 'The Duties Imposed by the Human Right to Basic Necessities', in T. Pogge (ed.), *Freedom From Poverty as a Human Right: Who Owes What to the Very Poor?* (Oxford: Oxford University Press, 2006).

[29] Putnam, *Bowling Alone*.

with social capital, and the dependence of the poor on it as a means to secure many benefits, it is important for the sake of justice that we be mindful of the impact of policy decisions on social capital. Indeed, a Rawlsian commitment to benefit the worst off might well dictate such a distribution.

The Obligation to Promote Social Capital: Ought Implies Can

To say that social capital is an ethical concept is also to assert something about its place among other normative goods. If I am right and there is a duty to promote social capital, then we ought to take it into account when we act both at individual and institutional levels. If social capital is a moral good, then it will need to be included in our moral deliberations about what actions we ought to perform, and what policies we ought to adopt. Moreover, to say that social capital is an ethical concept is to assign some responsibility for implementing it to those who work in the area of applied ethics, law, and public policy. Just as applied ethicists, lawyers, and judges consider the consequences of policies on individual liberty and autonomy, they should, arguably, do likewise for social capital. Some of this is already being done in countries such as Britain, Ireland, and Canada, where the impact of policy on a community's social capital is often considered. Applied ethicists, and social *and* political philosophers could do the same. They could begin to incorporate an analysis of the implications of policies on social capital reservoirs as a prerequisite to implementing those policies.

It makes little sense to identify the concept of social capital as an ethical concept, unless one can, at the same time, state upon whom the obligation to facilitate social capital would fall. Though I do not take up the question of whether there is a *right* to social capital in this paper, some of the problems that plague the so called 'manifesto rights' might well also plague a moral claim to social capital. On whom might the duty to provide social capital fall? The duty or obligation to cultivate social capital might fall on both individuals and institutions. Let's start with the easier case of individuals. Individuals might fulfill their obligations to cultivate social capital just as they do with many other obligations that they have: they ought to be mindful of the obligations in their daily interactions. When neighbours ask for small favours, such as watering the plants and feeding pets when on vacation, then social capital considerations might sway an otherwise ambivalent neighbour into one who would perform the favour. Similarly, joining civic organizations such as the Parents and Teachers Association, would be valuable not only because it would benefit your child, but also morally valuable because it would promote social capital for the community. There are countless instances when individuals can act in the service of social capital in their daily lives. The duty to facilitate social capital is likely to be a *prima facie* one.

Institutions, such as state and federal offices, non-governmental organizations and the judicial system, both local and international law, could also promote social capital. Organizing schedules and designing physical locations to facilitate interaction among people will be helpful. Courts that support community health will also contribute to social capital.[30] Enacting laws that encourage people to care for others, over those that don't, would promote social capital. Few jurisdictions in the US have enacted Good Samaritan laws. Failure to immunize people from legal repercussions in the event that when they render aid, and it goes amiss, discourages them from helping others. Such an omission might well change were one to incorporate a consideration of social capital in the decision about whether or not to enact Good Samaritan laws.[31]

Why Social Capital?

Social capital, generalized reciprocity, and the trust that enables them, have the potential to be important for global justice. Wealthy nations may be more willing to give to people in the developing world if social capital can be cultivated internationally. As Thomas Pogge has pointed out, people need to *care* about the object of human rights if we are ever to make progress toward realizing such rights.[32] Moreover, social capital is especially important because it enables other morally significant conduct, such as generosity, fairness (reciprocation), trustworthiness and philanthropy to name a few. The concept of generalized reciprocity seems especially relevant here since developing countries cannot reciprocate in kind. In a world rich in social capital, during times of public health crisis, at-risk countries such as China during the SARS scare, may be more willing to share politically incriminating information. Even if we know that ethically we have obligations to help those in the developing world,[33] we may require not only governmental, non-governmental and organizational help in order to fulfill these obligations, but also social capital. Social capital will both help people to 'own' their moral obligations to others, and to work with others to meet those obligations.

Some people may believe that the more lenient demands of generalized reciprocity may be excessive for those in the developing world. Arguably, developing countries cannot reciprocate at all. It is certainly true that people in the developing world cannot reciprocate in kind. But it is a mistake to assume that because they do not give in kind, they do not give at all. There is, for example, much documentation on the great exodus of nurses and nurse practitioners from

---

30 *Jacobson v Massachusetts Supreme Court* (1905).

31 R. Bhaskar and P. Illingworth, *Law, Economics, and Social Capital Formation* (forthcoming).

32 T. Pogge, *World Poverty and Human Rights* (Cambridge: Polity Press, 2002).

33 T. Pogge, '"Assisting" the Global Poor', in D.K. Chatterjee (ed.), *The Ethics of Assistance* (Cambridge: Cambridge University Press, 2004), pp. 260-88; P. Singer, *Practical Ethics* (Cambridge: Cambridge University Press, 1993).

developing countries to the developed world.[34] And of course, there is the use of sick and poor South Africans as research subjects in pharmaceutical trials for drugs that, in the end, most South Africans are unable to afford. Bioprospecting and biopiracy are two other examples in which often developing countries 'give' to wealthy nations.

As important for global justice as global social capital would be, however, there appear to be significant obstacles to achieving it. Most notably, ethnic and religious diversity appear to have an adverse effect on social capital. Studies have shown that social capital does not do well in heterogeneous communities. According to these studies, diversity impairs trust and social capital. If it is the case that diversity undermines social capital, the possibility of cultivating global social capital would be slim. It is, however, unlikely that the diversity problem is an insurmountable one. Building global social capital will require efforts to develop bridging social capital and to create the sorts of values, networks, and contacts that will allow social capital to transcend particular communities. Reported contact and exposure to people from other religious and ethnic communities can be helpful here. Homogenous communities may have to forfeit some of their social capital for the sake of enhancing the social capital of the global community. But if global social capital will secure some of the global goods I have suggested (such as reducing global poverty and disease), then it may well be worth the sacrifice in terms of increased benefits for all and the realization of human rights.

The evidence that diversity is bad for social capital comes primarily from economists. It shows that civic engagement (which, according to Putnam, is an important index of social capital) is lower in heterogeneous communities. Put differently, it appears that homogeneity enhances civic participation.[35] Costa and Khan provide the following explanation:

> Diversity … imposes costs. Whether in choosing a college roommate, a residential community, or a place to pray, people tend to self-segregate. They prefer to interact with others like them because of shared interests, socialization to the same cultural norms, and greater empathy toward individuals who remind them of themselves ….[36]

Implicit in the concept of social capital is the idea that relationships among people are good. But there is a dark side to social capital. When individuals are involved in their communities and communities are cohesive—when people interact with kindness and reciprocation, and are mindful of each other's interests—they may

---

[34] WHO (World Health Organization), *International Nurse Mobility: Trends and Implications* (Geneva: WHO, 2003). Available at: http://whqlibdoc.who.int/hq/2003/WHO_EIP_OSD_2003.3.pdf (accessed 13 June 2006).

[35] D.L. Costa and M.E. Khan, 'Civic Engagement and Community Heterogeneity: An Economist's Perspective', *Perspectives on Politics*, 1 (2003): 103-11.

[36] Ibid.

also exclude those who are not members of the community. Social capital creates an environment in which people are willing to act for the sake of others, even though they may not benefit immediately—they trust that the others will reciprocate at some later time because they *identify* with those others, and trust them.

It is perfectly understandable, though not necessarily rational, that people are drawn to those whom they perceive to be similar. There may appear to be safety in similarity. In the case of social capital, trust and social capital are enhanced when there are frequent face-to-face interactions. Given this and the preference to be with people who are similar to oneself, it is not surprising that social capital flourishes in homogenous communities. It is, after all, within those communities that people have face-to-face interactions. But surely in a global world it is not impossible to encourage face-to-face interactions among diverse people and populations?

I can only hint at some strategies that might be helpful in building a global fund of social capital. As we saw from the definitions and descriptions of social capital, norms and values are an important component of social capital. Creating global social capital, to be used in a global world where information is to be shared and wealthy nations are to give to poor ones, will require a paradigm shift—one that embraces the values of ethical and cultural cosmopolitanism in which individuals (not nations) are the relevant category.[37] [38]

As the global world becomes smaller, both through frequent travel for business and leisure, as well as widespread Internet and telecommunication use, people from diverse communities will have more frequent interactions. Moreover, as we come to understand our shared humanity—for example, through our shared vulnerability to contagions such as HIV, SARS and avian flu—we can anticipate greater trust between diverse communities. Increased travel and internet use may enhance interactions among people from diverse communities, but social capital is also enhanced by values and norms. It is not surprising that 'global social capital' is low when the dominant cultural and ethical values stress the importance, both culturally and morally, of acting for the benefit of those close, including family, friends, and compatriots. Although there are many good arguments that support cosmopolitanism, the need for increased social capital is another one. Support of cosmopolitan values, combined with various other measures that increase face-to-face contact with diverse people, may be fruitful for increasing global social capital, and in turn, global justice.[39]

37 T. Pogge, *World Poverty and Human Rights*; S. Scheffler, 'Conceptions of Cosmopolitanism', *Utilitas*, 11/3 (1999): 255-76.

38 S. Benatar, A. Darr and P. Singer, 'Global Health Ethics: the Rationale for Mutual Caring', *Internal Affairs*, 79/1 (2003): 107-38.

39 I wish to thank Solomon Benatar, Angus Dawson, Chris Megone, Wendy Parmet, Thomas Pogge, Rebecca Shah, John Tasioulas, and Dan Wikler for helpful comments on an earlier draft.

Chapter 5

On the Evaluative Space for Measuring Public Health Performance

Onyebuchi A. Arah
University of Amsterdam, National Institute of Public Health and the Environment, Netherlands and UCLA, USA

Current measurement systems for evaluating public health performance emphasize some essential functions derived from: emphasis on collective responsibility and role of the state, focus on whole populations, emphasis on prevention, concern for the underlying socio-economic determinants of health and disease, multi-disciplinary approach (both quantitatively and qualitatively), and partnerships with populations served. This functions-based approach or any other performance evaluation system must acknowledge what I describe as the two meanings of public health: the *health of the public* (which presents the *aggregative population* or 'ends perspective') or the *public of health* (which presents the *modus operandi* or 'means perspective'). I argue that an integrated approach which refocuses public health as both a *means* and an *end* is necessary for understanding how to measure its performance *vis-à-vis* what individuals and society may have reason to value in public health. Indeed, the evaluative space for measuring public health performance consists precisely in the extent to which public health provides and distributes *opportunities* for and secures actual *attainments* of health within the collective. In this new framework, individuals within the collective retain the *freedom* to gain from functional public health.

The topic of health system performance commands considerable attention among policymakers and academics worldwide. It has understandably become commonplace for countries to assess and 'incentivize' healthcare performance. International organizations such as the World Health Organization (WHO) and the Organisation for Economic Co-operation and Development (OECD) have taken a lead in encouraging health system performance measurement. The reasons for the increased interests are well-known: rising costs, technological advancements, aging populations, health market failures, poor quality and variations in practice, medical errors and injuries, lack of accountability, and inequalities among other things. These have led to widespread perceptions of poor value for the money and effort spent on healthcare. The latest efforts being made to manage the perennial problems of sub-optimal performance include the deployment of performance measurement, monitoring and improvement initiatives.[1] Many industrialized countries have, therefore, sought to manage 'health production' and their health goals through performance measurement.[2] However, the resulting performance measurement systems hardly pay attention to the role of public health in health system performance.[3] One reason is the lack of consensus about and poor appreciation of what public health means and does.[4] In some circles, public health is simply synonymous with preventive medicine and, sometimes unwittingly, with vaccination, and more recently, with health promotion to combat unhealthy lifestyles. To measure public health performance, we must first try to understand the meaning of public health.

Several years ago, the Acheson Report defined public health as 'the science and art of preventing disease, prolonging life, and promoting health through organized efforts of the society'.[5] Public health has, therefore, been seen as an alternative approach to personal medical care which has been taken to be very individualistic in its approach. The performance of public health may be judged almost exclusively in terms of this collective or non-individualistic approach. A close examination of current evaluative approaches to public health performance shows that the pillars for judging public health performance rest on some ten derivative essential functions that champion the 'collective' and are themselves products of the so-called principles of public health. These principles supposedly reflect the meaning and purpose of public health. In this paper, I will show that there are at least two meanings or perspectives of public health, both of which can easily be used to justify the *collective*: (1) the 'health of the public' (which presents the *aggregative population* or ends perspective) and (2) the 'public of health' (which presents the *modus operandi* or means perspective).

An *individualistic* (or 'the sum of the parts') interpretation of public health as against a *collective*[6] (or 'larger than the sum of the parts' or indivisible societal)

---

1 O.A. Arah, N.S. Klazinga, D.M.J. Delnoij, A.H.A. ten Asbroek, and T. Custers, 'Conceptual Frameworks for Health Systems Performance: A Quest for Effectiveness, Quality, and Improvement', *International Journal for Quality in Health Care*, 15/5 (2003): 377-98.

2 O.A. Arah, G.P. Westert, J. Hurst, and N.S. Klazinga. 'A Conceptual Framework for the OECD Health Care Quality Indicators Project', *International Journal for Quality in Health Care*, 18/Supplement 1 (2006): 5-13.

3 O.A. Arah, *Performance Reexamined. Concepts, Content and Practice of Measuring Health System Performance* (Amsterdam: Buijten & Schipperheijn Publishing and University of Amsterdam, Academic Medical Center, 2005): 21-82, 195-222.

4 Arah, *Peformance Reexamined.*

5 D. Acheson, *Public Health in England. The Report of the Committee of Inquiry into the Future Development of the Public Health Function* (London: HMSO, 1988).

6 A collective is a group of people who share or are motivated by at least one common issue or interest, or work together to achieve a common objective. See http://en.wikipedia.org/wiki/Collective (accessed 1 October, 2006).

interpretation of public health functioning, delivery mode, monitoring and subsequent performance measurement may be counterproductive. These somewhat mutually exclusive interpretations further worsen the existing tension between the individualistic focus of medical care and the collective purview of public health. Consequently, in measuring health and healthcare performance, where healthcare is the totality of medical care and public health, we often neglect the valuable contributions of public health.

In this paper, I argue that an integrated approach which refocuses public health as both a means and an end is necessary for understanding how to measure its performance *vis-à-vis* what individuals and society may have reason to value in public health. I will argue that the evaluative space for measuring public health performance consists precisely in the extent to which it provides and distributes *opportunities* for or actual *attainments* of health within the collective. In this new perspective, individuals within the collective retain the *freedom* to gain from functional public health, irrespective of whether they actually end up gaining or not. Relaxing the requirements for evaluating public health in this combined *opportunities*-and-*attainments* perspective may reduce the tension between the individual and the collective.

The outline of this paper is as follows: I first introduce the two meanings of public health.[7] Subsequently, I briefly address the question 'performance of what—and to what ends?',[8] showing how the answer can change the way we view the evaluative space for measuring public health performance, if not how we view public health as a discipline. Thereafter, I review how the current approach to assessing public health performance is based on ten functions grouped into three meta-functions derived from the so-called public health principles. Armed with the two meanings of public health which I will outline, I then propose a new evaluative space[9] that extends and revises the current functions-based performance system. By evaluative space, I mean the classificatory focus of measuring and valuing how well public health does in carrying out its functions in order to achieve its goal(s).

---

[7] Here, I take healthcare to mean *medical care* plus *public health*.

[8] This question draws our attention to the various claims public health can lay to health in terms of its role, functioning or performance. One must then wonder in what 'space' public health is defined and practiced. It has to be clear what this space is because it is in this space that we can judge whether public health is functional or not.

[9] It may be useful for the present discourse to think of public health performance evaluation as existing in some 'space' where we arbitrate public health functioning and attainments. It is in the choice of space that I pose the question 'performance of what—and to what ends?', an analogy that draws heavily from Amartya Sen's seminal work on the space of equality. See A.K. Sen, *Inequality Reexamined* (Oxford: Oxford University Press, 1992).

Two Meanings of Public Health

Before I contemplate the space in which public health performance should be evaluated, I must first address what public health is.[10] To understand what public health is,[11] I must look at what healthcare is and in particular at what medical care is. Going by what has become the most popular, succinct definition of public health—'the science and art of preventing disease, prolonging life, and promoting health through organized efforts of the society'[12]—I am inclined to see public health as the flip side of the healthcare coin. Surely, the whole of healthcare is concerned with 'preventing (future) disease, prolonging life, and promoting health'? Public health probably focuses more on prevention and promotion than medical care does. Of course, medical care deals with almost all of these things albeit in personal one-on-one interactions involving sick individuals and their physicians. Therefore, the difference between public health and personal medical care must lie in the phrase 'through the organized efforts of society'. Again, one can argue that organized efforts of society refers to almost all sectors of human endeavors including personal medical services as seen in clinics and hospitals at all levels of the healthcare system. However, such an argument will leave us with no distinction between public health and personal medical care. I prefer to see the phrase 'organized efforts of society' as portraying the collective mechanism or means by which public health is delivered and managed in a given society. This contrasts with the personal delivery mode of medical care. In other words, if medical care is the 'personal of health', then public health can be seen as the *public of health* or what I call the 'means perspective'.

There is yet another perspective to the meaning of public health, one that has been described as population health. This is described as 'the health outcomes of a group of individuals, including the distribution of such outcomes within the

[10] Since after presenting this paper at the conference of the Society for Applied Philosophy, I have been fortunate to receive and read Marcel Verweij and Angus Dawson's own stimulating contemporary analysis of the meaning of public health. It is interesting to see that we independently reached similar conclusions about the duality of the meaning public health. However, we differ on some nuanced but important interpretations of both the informational basis and consequences of this duality in the concept of public health; these differences will be the subject of another paper. See M. Verweij and A. Dawson, 'The Meaning of "Public" in Public Health', in Angus Dawson and Marcel Verweij (eds), *Ethics, Prevention and Public Health* (Oxford: Oxford University Press, 2007).

[11] Public health evokes many meanings, in particular two: (1) prevention and (2) organized or collective efforts of society. In this way, public health can be seen as the help which prevents a fall from the top of a cliff, while personal medical care may be seen as what Norman Daniels referred to as 'the ambulance at the bottom of the cliff after the free fall through life'.

[12] Acheson, *Public Health in England.*

group'.[13] This is what I describe as the *health of the public* or the 'ends perspective' to denote the health status attainments of and health distribution *within* the collective. I use the term 'collective' to denote a self-sufficient group of individuals who share a common characteristic or goal. This collective is difficult to understand by looking at the sum of isolated individual members. This interpretation of the ends perspective complements the collective means of public health delivery and actions.

Therefore, public health is perhaps best described as the science and art of collectively preventing disease, prolonging life, and promoting the levels and distributions of health in a society. This does not tell us much about the place of the autonomous individual members of the society. It would seem as if in the pursuit of the common good we could be willing to sacrifice individual freedom, an enduring source of tension between the personal focus of medical care and the collective purview of public health. According to John Stuart Mill,[14] every individual in a democracy must have the freedom to live the way she chooses insofar as she does not harm another in the process. Ultimately, public health is, as Jean Foster argues, fundamentally about community and about the shared values of life, health, and security.[15]

Performance of What—and to What Ends?

I have argued elsewhere[16] that any evaluation of performance must begin with the question 'performance of what—and to what ends?'.[17] In all performance evaluation systems, performance or functioning is linked to at least one core goal. I argue that practically all performance measurement systems aim at evaluating the performance of *something* that public health is supposed to be doing for societies, often relating to a specific goal or group of goals such as addressing population health needs, risks, or inequalities. The space in which that goal is evaluated can differ according to the approach used to attain the goal in question. In the case of medical care, the answer to the question lies in the performance of

---

[13] D. Kindig and G. Stoddart, 'What is Population Health?, *American Journal of Public Health*, 93/3, (2003): 380-83.

[14] John Stuart Mill, *On Liberty* (New York: Penguin Books, 1975 (1859)).

[15] See D.E. Beauchamp, 'What is Public about Public Health?', *Health Affairs*, 2/4 (1983): 76-87.

[16] Arah, *Performance Reexamined.*

[17] For a similar line of reasoning in welfare economics and philosophy, see A.K. Sen, 'Equality of What?' in S. M. McMurrin (ed.), Tanner Lectures on Human Values (Salt Lake City: University of Utah Press and Cambridge: Cambridge University Press, 1980) and Sen, Inequality Reexamined. See also M. Nussbaum, Frontiers of Justice: Disability, Nationality, Species Membership (The Tanner Lectures in Human Values), (Cambridge, MA: Belknap Press of Harvard University, 2006).

personal delivery of medical care to attain health in individual patients. Given the arguments for the collective means and ends interpretation of public health, the performance of public health must then be seen as the functioning of its collective means and ends.

The importance of the question 'performance of what—and to what ends?' derives from the actual variety in the substantive goals of public health. This variety is evident in the abovementioned functions and principles of public health. Thus, it makes sense that each function demands a certain performance of something that public health must deliver, be it setting priorities for population health or assuring the quality of public health policies aimed at maintaining health or combating negative effects of health determinants. This richness and diversity in the focal interests of public health are of such substantive importance that they are primary or foundational—*not secondary*—to our interest in measuring public health performance.

The diversity in public health functions—and therefore, performance—represents the various health needs of societies and the variety of health determinants that are socially patterned. But why the collective approach?

There are several important reasons for the collective means and mechanism of public health. Firstly, in any given collective, a collective approach would be inevitable whenever the causal effect of a determinant is probabilistic even within a partially deterministic causal system. It may be difficult, if not impossible, to identify specific individuals who would certainly be at risk of ill-health and could therefore gain from early intervention. For example, although we know from epidemiology that cigarette smoking causes lung cancer among a host of other illnesses, we cannot tell exactly who among smokers will actually end up having cancer and when, simply because smoking does not always cause lung cancer in all smokers. Here, we must resort to some form of anti-smoking intervention or tobacco control at the whole (relevant for all smokers) population level.

Secondly, many determinants of health are behavioural in nature and are often socially conditioned, making it sometimes impossible for public health to influence such determinants within a collective environment where the conditioning of individual choices and actions occurs.

Thirdly, we must also choose the collective approach whenever this is the only feasible way of delivering the intervention in question, for example, fluoridation of water supplies.

Fourthly, epidemiological evidence tells us that when many people within the collective receive small benefits, the total collective benefit (that is, the population-wide gain) may actually be large.[18]

Fifthly, the collective approach is also justified whenever we are interested in the distal causes of disease or the causes of causes, such as the social, economic, and political determinants of health and ill-health.

---

[18] G. Rose, *The Strategy of Preventive Medicine* (Oxford: Oxford University Press, 1992).

Sixthly, the collective approach is appropriate for contextualizing the individual interests and rights which political association is designed to protect; it also defines the individual as part of a political community which, despite diversity and pluralism, is more than the sum of the private interests. As a member of a collective, an individual is subject to laws and regulations designed to advance the common good.

From Principles to Functions: Current Public Health Performance Assessment

Public health practitioners and researchers happily point out that there are some core binding, albeit overlapping, principles which define public health as a specialty, a scientific endeavour, and a social commitment to health. These principles which were mostly developed during the 1990s are:[19]

- emphasis on collective responsibility and the role of the state
- focus on whole populations
- emphasis on prevention
- concern for the underlying socioeconomic determinants of health and disease
- multi-disciplinary approach (both quantitatively and qualitatively) and
- partnerships with populations served.

The first principle tells us that public health lays emphasis on collective responsibility for health, in particular one that requires an active governmental role.[20] The second principle stipulates that the focus should be on whole populations: in a sense, we could interpret this as meaning that under certain conditions an individual's priorities must be subsumed under the collective goal. For instance, when we vaccinate to attain herd immunity we do so for the common good. The third principle promotes the idea of prevention, that is, the avoidance of disease, ill-health or disability. This principle cannot, however, be construed as implying a collective goal or not, unless we are willing to accept that what is being prevented is, by definition, socially or collectively patterned. Nonetheless, a closer look at current practices leads us to think that public health practitioners see prevention as a *collectively* delivered *common* goal.

The fourth principle points out that public health must deal with the socioeconomic determinants of health and disease, perhaps buttressing the

---

19 C.A. Miller, K.S. Moore, T.B. Richards, and J.D. Monk, 'A Proposed Method for Assessing the Performance of Local Public Health Functions and Practices', *American Journal of Public Health*, 84/11 (1994): 1743-9.

20 For an illuminating discussion on the strengths and weaknesses of requiring the government's role as an interpretation of the collective approach to delivering public health, see Verweij and Dawson, 'The Meaning of "Public" in Public Health'.

collective mechanism and the collective goal. The collective mechanism here has to do with the fact that socioeconomic factors are socially patterned. Their removal or prevention appears to lie in the collective. An under-appreciated aspect of this fourth principle is its focus on not only disease but also health.

The fifth principle is a research-related one: public health should embrace all research methods. Unfortunately, this principle presupposes that there are two worlds of research methods, namely, qualitative and quantitative. We might suspect that the architects of this principle think that there are soft and hard approaches to research. We can only question why this should be a principle of public health.

The sixth and final principle addresses the need for partnering with the populations served in order to attain population health goals. Probably, this is what the Acheson Commission, just like Winslow,[21] might have meant by 'organized efforts of society'.[22] Much like the first, second and fourth, this principle emphasizes the collective, this time by focusing on the mechanism of public health functioning (that is, the 'public of health' or the *means perspective* described earlier).

Taken together, these principles have been used over time to justify ten *functions* or practices of public health.[23] These functions are further grouped into three so-called meta-functions—namely, assessment, policy development, and assurance.[24]

Assessment:

- assessing the health needs of the community
- investigating the occurrence of health effects and health hazards in the community
- analyzing the determinants of identified health needs.

Policy Development:

- advocating for public health, building constituencies, and identifying resources in the community
- setting priorities among health needs
- developing plans and policies to address priority health needs.

Assurance:

- managing resources and developing organizational structure
- implementing programmes

[21] C.E.A. Winslow, 'The Untilled Fields of Public Health', *Science*, 51 (1920): 23.

[22] Acheson, *Public Health in England.*

[23] Miller et al., 'A Proposed Method'.

[24] The Institute of Medicine, *The Future of Public Health* (Washington DC: National Academies Press, 1988).

- evaluating programmes and providing quality assurance
- informing and educating the public.

Again, the collective approach is noticeable in these functions. One gets the feeling that public health is largely concerned with the collective determination, identification, consequences and solution of health issues in a society. Nonetheless, these functions do not necessarily point out what constitutes an evaluative space for measuring public health performance.

Towards an Evaluative Space for Measuring Public Health Performance

Assessing a society's and its individual members' capabilities or opportunities to attain health provides a useful general approach to evaluating public health performance. Indeed, the evaluative space for measuring public health performance consists of the extent to which public health provides *opportunities or freedom to attain health within the collective*, and the actual *attainment of health levels and distributions* that a society and its members have reason to value. I call this evaluative space the *opportunities-and-attainment* approach. This is in line with Amartya Sen's capability approach to evaluating welfare, development and justice. Sen describes his capability approach as follows: *capability* refers to the *extent* of the sets of *freedom to achieve* things we have reason to value; *functioning* refers to the level of actual *achievements*. Sen uses his capability theory as a general approach to viewing and assessing social arrangements. This approach can be traced back to Aristotelian traditions.[25]

For an extension of the capability approach to work here, I view public health as a specific kind of social arrangement and I have already argued the case for this in the preceding sections of this paper. The identification of the goals of the value objects of public health allows for the specification of the *evaluative space* for measuring public health performance.

However, there are a series of (additional) important observations and arguments that help justify the evaluative space in which to measure public health performance. These observations are as follows:

- Health is a complex product of the complex *causal* interactions of at least four categories of determinants, namely—genes or host biology, environment, lifestyle, and healthcare.
- Three of these are largely socially patterned (read: can be subsumed under the collective): environment, lifestyle, and healthcare.
- Healthcare can influence all the other determinants either at the collective (public health) or individual (personal medical care) level.
- It is difficult to understand the health effects of healthcare without

[25] A.K. Sen, *Commodities and Capabilities* (Amsterdam: North Holland, 1985).

understanding the effects of the other determinants, especially the impact of healthcare on these other factors.

- Public health performance must be seen in terms of how public health functions in influencing health via the usually socially patterned non-healthcare determinants.
- Since there are non-healthcare determinants which are socially patterned and which are rarely ever seen as individual-level features but as collective dynamics, then public health performance must also be seen as a collective mechanism (means perspective for the *extent of opportunities* to benefit from public health) for a collective goal (*population health attainment* within the ends perspective). In other words, the demands of the new evaluative space for public health performance must be seen within the context of the causal determinants of health and the levels and distribution of the burden of these determinants and their health effects in any given society.

Irrespective of whether everyone actually benefits and allowing for some degree of individual choice of non-participation, public health performance can be assessed in terms of the *extent of opportunities* to benefit from a collectively provided health-yielding intervention within a collective.[26] An intervention can only be seen as a public health success if, and only if, it is a means of delivering a public health intervention that increases the propensity to benefit individual members who otherwise would suffer the negative effects of not consuming that intervention. My argument allows room for individuals to opt out of participating in the intervention only to the extent that their non-participation does not put others at risk.

This interpretation of the *means* perspective of public health in the *extent of opportunities* or effective freedom[27] it provides could run into a grey area if passive benefits or side-effects of a population-level intervention would nonetheless reach non-consenting individuals. This may arise when a public health problem has a high externality factor, that is, it affects other 'proximate' members of the collective who are at risk of some form of ill-health in the absence of intervention. In this scenario, it would be difficult to defend whether a remedial population-level intervention would not have been implemented intentionally in such a way as to benefit even non-consenting individuals for their own good. This could easily be the case in aggressive vaccination campaigns which conferred herd immunity and which would unusually and deliberately be targeted at enough consenting persons in order to achieve herd immunity anyway in mixed communities of consenting

26 The term *collective* leaves the unsavoury taste of simplistic aggregation, yet it has a powerful way of reminding us that every society or collective is made up of individuals who are bound in the rich tapestry of some common good.

27 Effective freedom implies that the opportunities to benefit need not be under the direct control of the beneficiary but satisfies the requirement that the opportunities take the form of what we value and want, or what we *would* choose *vis-à-vis* our objectives.

and non-consenting members. Hence, public health may not always be able to guarantee effective freedom or opportunities to benefit (or to opt out) when a population-level intervention has beneficial 'side-effects' for non-participants.

When public health succeeds in removing barriers to meaningful enjoyment of the benefits of available interventions, we may say public health is performing well. For example, freedom of obtaining and accessing balanced information, vaccines, transportation to vaccination centres, and freedom of thought and informed choice are some of the important indicators of the opportunities space for evaluating public health performance for vaccinations. How good such performance could be is a matter I will not pursue further here because an assessment of the *value* of attained performance is beyond the scope of this paper.

The *extent* of the opportunities to benefit from public health must be distinguished from the *means* of achieving such opportunities. For example, the number or rate of vaccinations administered by school programmes or general practice contacts in a society represent the means of conferring immunity but need not represent the extent of immunity actually conferred, a parameter that is dependent on a number of other related factors such as the ability of individual members of the society to seroconvert the vaccines given. Two different societies might have the same vaccination rates but different immunity levels, and therefore potentially differing levels of protection against the disease in question. Their individual members might even have different opportunities for gaining from vaccination campaigns and/or from the conferrable immunity. In other words, there is an important philosophical, if not practical, difference in the *resources that help* us to attain opportunities to gain from public health and *the extent of such opportunities*. Opportunities have to be distinguished not just from attainments, but also from the resources and means to opportunities. Interpersonal and social characteristics within any collective can lead to substantial interpersonal and social variations in the conversion of resources and means into health attainments. Likewise, such characteristics can also lead to variations in the conversion of resources and means into real opportunities[28] to attain health.

Assuring the freedom to enjoy public health measures that one may have reason to value can be paired with what attainments or ends such a freedom should lead to. It is quite possible, however, to envisage the attainment of health without paying too much attention to the range of opportunities from which individuals and society choose in order to attain their current and future levels and distribution of health. It is easy to see that population health, that is the health status levels and distributions within the collective, must be firmly dependent on the nature of the collective health attainments. One might still wonder, how do *opportunities*—as opposed to actual health attainments—relate to population health?

The connection between opportunities to attain and population health is two-fold. First, if attained health constitutes population health, then the opportunities to

[28] Sen, *Inequality Reexamined.* See also A.K. Sen, *Commodities and Capabilities* (Amsterdam: North Holland, 1985).

attain health will constitute the freedom or real opportunities to achieve population health. This freedom, reflecting the collective's opportunities for population health must be valued at least for *instrumental reasons*, for example in evaluating how good a public health fortune the collective has in the universe of collectives. On the other hand, enjoying the opportunities to attain health may be valued for its sake, in being an intrinsically valuable or good social structure in and of itself. A good society is also a society of freedom, including the opportunities to attain the population health it has reason to value.[29] Here, John Rawls[30] and his proponents may prefer to see these opportunities as *rightness* as opposed to *goodness* in arguing for the priority of *right* over ideas of the *good*. However, this interesting perspective on the first connection between opportunities and attained population health is beyond the scope of this paper.

The second connection between opportunities and population health lies in making *attained* population health itself depend on the *opportunities* to attain. In some respects, some types of opportunities (say, herd immunity) contribute directly to population health. The real range of opportunities provides information on the different population health attainments that are within the reach of a collective, and this information is crucial, irrespective of how precisely population health is described.

This new evaluative space differs from current public health performance approaches that tend to emphasize organizational functions of public health and therefore the provision of resources for health (and which, for instance, track immunization rates as opposed to seroconversion or actual disease prevention rates). Such functions-based assessments tend to be overly concerned with the means or *instruments* of attaining public health functioning. On the other hand, *opportunities to attain health* and *actual health attainments* are constitutive of and conducive to population health.

Conclusions

In this paper, I have tried to outline concepts that should guide the development of the evaluative space for measuring public health performance. I have argued that the diversity of goals of public health imply that we must always begin the evaluative exercise by addressing the question 'performance of what—and to what ends?' in order to centralize the goals being targeted and valued. To manage the plurality of public health goals, I presented at least two broad meanings of public health that highlight the means and ends of public health as being foundational to its meaning, purview and functioning. This clarification supports an opportunities-and-attainments evaluative space for measuring public health performance.

29 Sen, *Inequality Reexamined.*

30 J. Rawls, *A Theory of Justice* (Cambridge, MA: Belknap Press of Harvard University Press, 1971).

The opportunities-and-attainments space readily complements the collective *means* and *ends* meanings of public health. This new evaluative approach allows for modification of the prevailing functions-based performance approach which has strong organizational leanings. On a closing note, if we side with Margaret Thatcher in arguing that there is no such thing as society, then we have no business discussing the philosophy of public health. The philosophy of public health is indeed the philosophy of society where society must be seen as being more than a mere aggregate of its individual members.

Chapter 6
Global Concerns and Local Arguments: How a Localized Bioethics may Perpetuate Injustice

Søren Holm
Cardiff University, UK and University of Oslo, Norway

In this paper I will consider to what extent a globalization of bioethics can be justified and what the likely negative side-effects of such a globalization may be. I will suggest that there are many instances where what is taking place under the name of globalization is not a true globalization of bioethics, but instead a spread of what the legal theorist Bonaventura de Sousa Santos has called 'globalized localisms', the introduction of specific institutional arrangements and value systems indigenous to western culture, across the globe.[1] I will argue for four main conclusions:

1. That for those, who like myself are objectivists or realists in moral theory, globalization of ethics is a natural goal, but that how this goal should be pursued does not follow in any straightforward way from those theoretical commitments.
2. That there is a need to distinguish sharply between globalizing ethics and globalizing specific institutional forms of ethics governance.
3. That our thinking concerning institutional forms of ethics governance has to be considerably more sensitive to the way in which the historical development of these institutions has shaped them.
4. That discussion of a global bioethics needs to be much more sensitive to the large differences in background conditions in different parts of the world.

The first part of this paper is mainly theoretical, whereas the second part is more practical. In this paper I am not discussing the issue of whether bioethics as an academic field is truly a global endeavour in its concerns, arguments or

---

[1] B de S Santos, *Towards a New Common Sense: Law, Science and Politics in the Paradigmatic Transition* (New York: Routledge, 1995).

institutional structure, but readers interested in that question can consult Holm & Williams-Jones (2006) and the references in that paper.[2]

From Objectivism to Globalization

Let us for the sake of argument assume the following to be true: (1) there are objective and universally applicable ethical values or principles[3], (2) these can in principle be known by humans and (3) they are of such a level of generality that (strong) particularism is false.

From this, combined with the premise that we ought to act morally, it follows that we have compelling reasons to try to elucidate what these values or principles are, to act in accordance with them, and to try to influence others to understand the values and principles and act in accordance with them. For objectivist, non-particularists like myself the globalization of ethics is thus a natural and morally required goal.

But the second premise only guarantees that the ethical values can be known, it does not guarantee that they are easily known, or that they are actually currently known by anyone. Even the simplest ethical systems are under continual modification and refinement (e.g. the journal *Utilitas* is still going strong), and we still lack agreement, even among objectivists on very basic questions concerning the structure of ethical systems. Our current ethical systems are therefore, at most, reasonably well corroborated hypotheses concerning the shape and content of the correct, justified and coherent system. It still makes sense to try to globalize our best current hypothesis, but this will have to be done in a tentative way, accepting that certain elements will change in the future.[4] As an initial consideration this ought to inspire a certain humility in our globalization attempts. Scepticism about a certain strong version of the globalization of ethics does therefore not necessarily imply moral relativism or nihilism, but just something that we might call moral fallibilism. The realization that whereas our current moral understanding is the best we have, it is not certain and almost certainly revisable in the future. It can be promoted as the best way forward, but not as the Truth about morality (capital 'T' intended).

---

2 S. Holm and B. Williams-Jones, 'Global Bioethics—Myth or Reality?', *BMC Medical Ethics*, 7/10 (2006) doi:10.1186/1472-6939-7-10 http://www.biomedcentral.com/1472-6939/7/10

3 Nothing in the argument to follow hinges on whether we are talking about values, principles, theories, systems, frameworks etc. or whether we prefer to label such an approach objectivist or realist.

4 Here we might note that at least some people are more certain about some particular judgements than about the precise justification for those judgements.

Human Rights as the Basic Minimum

But could we not argue that human rights as specified in declarations and conventions form a solid basis for globalizing bioethics and that they are actually fixed?[5] They have furthermore been freely accepted by the states that are signatories to the documents, and they are held to be deducible from our objective ethical principles.

While such an argument is tempting it is also problematic. It is first not clear that all the human rights enunciated in even the most authoritative documents are uncontroversially deducible from ethical theory. A standard example of this is Article 24 in the *Universal Declaration of Human Rights* (1948), arguably the most authoritative document of its kind:

'Everyone has the right to rest and leisure, including reasonable limitation of working hours and periodic holidays with pay'.

The first part of this Article probably does describe a human right that is deducible from any plausible moral theory, but can we really deduce a right to 'periodic holidays with pay' from ethical theory in any straightforward manner? Getting such a right from for instance consequentialism, libertarianism or a principlist approach will require significant argumentative contortions.

But maybe there is a set of uncontroversially deducible human rights we can rely on, the core set. However, even if we are not Benthamite sceptics concerning the very existence of human rights we will still have to recognize that (1) there will be disagreement concerning the exclusion and inclusion of specific rights in the uncontroversial, core set and (2) that there will be disagreement concerning the exact meaning of the rights in the set.[6] To continue with Article 24 there is undoubtedly disagreement concerning what is 'reasonable limitation of working hours', and I know many university professors who work far more hours than, for instance, the legislators in the European Union think is reasonable (on average 48 hours a week as a maximum).[7]

---

[5] This would approximate a hyper-robust version of the human rights approach suggested by Jonathan Mann, 'Medicine and public health, ethics and human rights', *Hastings Center Report* 27/3 (1997): 6-13.

[6] J. Waldron, (ed.) *Nonsense Upon Stilts: Bentham, Burke and Marx on the Rights of Man*. (London: Routledge, 2007).

[7] Council Directive No. 93/104/EC of 23 November 1993 concerning certain aspects of the organization of working time. 'Article 6—Maximum weekly working time:

Member States shall take the measures necessary to ensure that, in keeping with the need to protect the safety and health of workers:

1. the period of weekly working time is limited by means of laws, regulations or administrative provisions or by collective agreements or agreements between the two sides of industry;

2. the average working time for each seven-day period, including overtime, does not exceed 48 hours'.

Second, the fixity of human rights is only a convenient legal fiction. The text may be fixed but its interpretation changes over time. It is rather obvious that Article 16 of the *Universal Declaration* is not interpreted in the same way now as it was in 1948, and that it is not interpreted in the same way by all signatories:

1. Men and women of full age, without any limitation due to race, nationality or religion, have the right to marry and to found a family. They are entitled to equal rights as to marriage, during marriage and at its dissolution.
2. Marriage shall be entered into only with the free and full consent of the intending spouses.
3. The family is the natural and fundamental group unit of society and is entitled to protection by society and the State.

In 1948 it was obvious that this article applied to heterosexual marriages only, but today some countries interpret it to apply to both heterosexual and homosexual marriages, whereas some other countries still prohibit homosexuality and consider the idea of homosexual marriage anathema.

These problems could indicate that it is preferable not to rely on the deducibility of the rights from ethical theory, but instead to rely exclusively on the agreement of the state parties involved. By their initial agreement they have accepted the existence of these rights and accepted to be bound by them, and by not withdrawing they have signalled their continued agreement.

But this argument is again largely based on legal fiction. Formal acceptance of the human rights documents is in many cases a condition for joining and continuing to be a member of certain organizations that most countries want to join and remain members of, for reasons totally unrelated to human rights. A member state of the European Union can, for instance not withdraw from the European Convention on Human Rights and still continue to be a member; and membership of the United Nations requires acceptance of the *Universal Declaration*.

This makes it doubtful whether we can imply any commitment to the contents of the documents, from the fact that they have been signed and ratified.[8] This does not mean that we cannot hold countries to their legal human rights commitments, but it does mean that we cannot imply that they have accepted these rights in more than the narrowest legal sense of accepting. We have no reason to believe that all states for instance endorse the right to 'periodic holidays with pay' or think that it is a truly justifiable human right universally applicable to all employees and all employers. So, whereas human rights and human rights discourse is undoubtedly important it does not provide us with an uncontroversial way of globalizing bioethics.

---

[8] As a parallel it is interesting to note that many ethicists have made the claim that the acceptance by third world countries of the World Trade Organization (WTO) *TRIPS Agreement* on IP protection can not be taken to imply true acceptance of the contents of this agreement, but is simply a reflection of both their desire to enter the WTO and their weak bargaining position.

Institutions, Political Philosophy and Compromise

If we look more closely at globalization initiatives within bioethics we see that they are often a curious mix of all kinds of different prescriptions and principles ranging from the very abstract level of ethical values and principles, to very specific prescriptions concerning procedures and institutions.

At one end of the spectrum we have attempts to globalize a specific, overarching ethical framework as the correct way to think about ethical issues in the bioethics field. At the other end we have very specific prescriptions concerning the content of patient information sheets and the constitution of research ethics committees in the context of biomedical research.

I will not say any more about the attempts to globalize ethical frameworks since as an objectivist, non-particularist I am myself committed to this kind of globalization with the caveat mentioned above.

There are, however, additional problems in globalizing bioethics procedures and institutions. One of the problems is that a specific institutional set-up often requires complicated trade-offs between different ethical considerations. In a recent paper in the *Journal of Medical Ethics*, Dawson and Garrard argue that this is not a problem since the agreements involve a commitment to the trade-off:

> International infectious disease prevention through the World Health Organization's (WHO's) regulations—for example, involves a commitment to agreement across the world about the trade-off between freedom of movement and the need to prevent the transmission of disease.[9]

But is this a correct inference from the fact that a set of regulations have been agreed? Let us first note that moral agreement comes in many forms. The Norwegian philosopher Knut Erik Tranøy has analyzed the concept of moral agreement and identified three different outcomes when two people discuss the morality of a proposition *p*:

1. Person A and B can agree that p is *unacceptable*, i.e. both mean *positively* that p should not be accepted,
2. A and B can agree that p is *acceptable*, i.e. both mean *positively* that p should be accepted,
3. A and B can agree that p is acceptable, but A or B might *abstain* from actively taking a stand on p.

---

[9] A. Dawson and E. Garrard, 'In defence of moral imperialism: four equal and universal prima facie principles', *Journal of Medical Ethics*, 32 (2006): 203.

Tranøy calls the last option 'open consensus'.[10] In a situation with many actors it becomes very likely that it is this last option that obtains, that agreement is reached not by positive commitment, but by some actors not taking a stand on the issue.

We also need to consider the process leading to such international regulations not as an exercise in moral reasoning, but as an exercise in negotiation and bargaining. In the specific case of the WHO regulations we have a bargaining situation where not reaching agreement has significant costs for everyone, for instance because it significantly complicates travel across borders. In such a bargaining situation each actor can be conceptualized as having an upper and a lower limit for what it sees as an acceptable trade-off between freedom of movement and the need to prevent the spread of infectious diseases (a bargaining range) and a preferred point within this bargaining range. As long as there is some overlap between these bargaining ranges an agreement can in principle be reached, although the exact point of the agreement may not be one that any actor would have specified as the ideal point. But in many bargaining situations an agreement is reached outside the initial bargaining range of some of the actors, because they are offered positive or negative incentives to move outside of their initial range. This may for instance be the case where most have reached an agreement, but a few actors still refuse to agree. In such a situation significant pressure may be applied to the recalcitrant few.

From the fact that agreement was reached, we can therefore only conclude that the trade-off was accepted (perhaps grudgingly) in the specific bargaining situation, and that no one found the trade-off so bad that they were willing to block an agreement, i.e. that it was not so far outside the bargaining range of one or more actors to be seen by them to be completely unacceptable.

What we can conclude from the fact of agreement is thus significantly less than Dawson and Garrard claim.

A further problem is that the regulations and institutions that are globalized often have a history, most often a history in the developed world. From the regulation it is clear that we are not sitting at the drawing board with a blank sheet of paper considering how, for instance research ethics should be regulated on a global scale. We are looking at 'tried and tested' models and tweaking them a little. We are thus proceeding in a way that is path-dependent and that will in many instances lead to a globalization of what are essentially localisms, i.e. institutional arrangements and ways of doing things that have developed in a local context (the commitment in Article 21 of the *Universal Declaration* to representative democracy could be seen as such a globalized localism. Although not much discussed today, there are numerous other options for non-authoritarian governance structures, anarcho-syndicalism was for instance an alternative much discussed in the 1930s;

10 K.E. Tranøy, *Det åpne sinn: moral og etikk mot et nytt årtusen [The open mind: morality and ethics towards a new millennium]* (Oslo: Universitetsforlaget, 1998). I owe the translation from Norwegian to Jan Helge Solbakk.

and even Rawls, a stalwart of liberalism accepts some forms of authoritarian rule as permissible in 'The Law of Peoples').[11]

Many principles of research ethics can best be understood by tracing them back to the origins of research ethics in the regulation of clinical research, and the ubiquity of the 'independent research ethics committee' as a necessary part of research ethics regulation can probably only be understood if we understand the history of the *Helsinki Declaration*, the history of the US Institutional Review Board system and the forces that shaped those histories. It is fairly obvious that if you introduce the device of a research ethics committee it should be 'independent' (however we interpret that requirement), but it is somewhat unclear exactly what independent means (independent of what and whom?), and much less obvious that a committee is the best governance structure.

Because western localisms are often already established and because they are the localisms of powerful actors on the international stage they are very likely to become globalized, because it will be difficult to persuade or force the holders of these localisms to give them up when negotiating for international agreement.

But there is clearly no reason to believe that, predominantly western localisms have any special claim to be globalized, and the more specific the features of the regulation or institutional set up, the less likely it is that there is any independent justification for globalizing these specific features.

Globalizing localisms may in many instances be innocuous (the research ethics committee is probably a case in point), but we have no reason to believe that this is always the case. For instance attempting to globalize the chaotic localism of the US healthcare system would arguably be a major disaster.[12]

Can we identify any problematic or potentially problematic bioethics globalized localisms at the institutional or regulatory level?

Recently some have claimed that the prohibition of trade in human organs, the injunction against reproductive cloning, or the blanket ban on doping in sport fall in to this category, but since I personally tend to believe that all of these are, at least potentially, justifiable I will instead focus on the requirement to establish clinical ethics committees found in Article 19.b of the recent UNESCO *Universal Declaration on Bioethics and Human Rights*:

> 'Article 19—Ethics committees
>
> Independent, multidisciplinary and pluralist ethics committees should be established, promoted and supported at the appropriate level in order to:

[11] J. Rawls, *The Law of Peoples* (Cambridge, MA: Harvard University Press, 1999).

[12] The ethical debate concerning the global trade system is also to a large extent a debate about the deleterious effects of globalized localisms and of various more or less radical proposals to abolish or significantly alter them. The intellectual property system is, for instance, not 'natural' but a specific institutional design suitable for late industrial societies.

(a) assess the relevant ethical, legal, scientific and social issues related to research projects involving human beings;
(b) provide advice on ethical problems in clinical settings;
(c) assess scientific and technological developments, formulate recommendations and contribute to the preparation of guidelines on issues within the scope of this Declaration;
(d) foster debate, education and public awareness of, and engagement in, bioethics'.

The requirement to introduce clinical ethics committees is clearly a globalized localism, few countries have them as yet and they mostly exist in the richer parts of the world. What is potentially problematic about this? First, it is far from clear that clinical ethics committees are actually the best way to solve ethical problems in clinical settings or whether, if you want to introduce ethics support, they are the most appropriate mechanism, even in those countries where they already exist. Second, it is not at all obvious that many of the ethical problems that necessarily arise in a significantly under-funded healthcare system can or should be dealt with by a committee, even an independent, multidisciplinary and pluralist committee. If the most basic problem is that there are not sufficient resources to provide even minimally adequate care for all who need it, the problem seems to be located at a very different level, and using resources on a clinical ethics committee seems ill-advised.

The Globalization of Respect for Autonomy

Let us finally consider the globalization of respect for autonomy and its potential negative effects on justice and wellbeing. I have chosen this example because I believe that respect for autonomy is one of the main contenders for a universal ethical principle and that it is part of any plausible ethical system. It is only an example and a similar analysis could be performed for other principles, values or virtues. I do not believe that respect for autonomy takes precedence over other principles, values or virtues, but it does provide a nice exemplar for the thesis that globalization often involves the globalization of localisms.

Respect for autonomy plays a role in many areas of bioethics including research ethics, public health ethics, reproductive ethics, the organization of the healthcare system and the trade in tissues and organs. In some of these areas it is mainly used in arguments to protect individuals from state intervention or from (involuntary) exploitation by powerful groups (e.g. medical researchers), and in other areas it is used to protect individuals from state or societal restrictions on their activities.[13],[14]

Globalizing respect for autonomy as an important ethical principle is thus, as far as I can see, warranted. We may well continue our discussions concerning exactly how important autonomy is in comparison to the other things that we value, but as long as we are sensitive to those complications we should be able to go ahead and promote respect for autonomy on a global scale.

But globalizing bioethicists are usually not content with globalizing ethical frameworks, they also want to globalize specific answers to specific ethical problems, and this is where I think the globalizing zeal often goes wrong, by neglecting the huge differences in background conditions around the world. We can imagine a context-sensitive globalization of respect for autonomy and perhaps even describe what this would entail in principle, but I think it is incontrovertible that most globalization attempts are not (sufficiently) context-sensitive.

Within a Western European context we can, for instance, assume background conditions including a relatively well-ordered society under the rule of law, significant regulation of the activities of commercial actors, reasonably effective legal enforcement, relatively well-educated actors, almost complete absence of abject poverty, limited inequalities between men and women etc. But this set of background factors cannot be assumed globally. Most people live under conditions that are vastly different from the conditions in Western Europe. This means that not all removals of government constraints on individual actions that enhance opportunities in Western Europe are likely to enhance opportunities everywhere, for instance, because they are only opportunity-enhancing (all things considered) if the actions of powerful commercial actors are efficiently-regulated, or because those who seemingly make use of the new opportunity are forced to do it.[15]

Another possible side-effect of promoting personal autonomy that is not very important in countries with well-functioning welfare systems is the effect on family cohesion. If the promotion of personal autonomy reduces family cohesion

[13] Let me before my critical comments just state for the record that I am in no doubt that we need more respect for autonomy and not less, but this does not detract from the fact that certain aspects of the globalization of respect for autonomy are problematic.

[14] In the present context I will not analyze the complicated relation between respect for personal autonomy and respect for the liberty of purely legal persons (companies, trusts etc.).

[15] It is often argued that we have no justification for intrusive questioning concerning why people choose to avail themselves of a medical intervention, as long as it is legal. But this means that in societies where at least some people are likely to be forced to ask for these interventions, we have no way of protecting them, except through a long term change of culture. It is no coincidence that most kidneys sold by live 'donors' in India come from women, and it would also be naïve to believe that all women who choose to have an abortion after determination of the sex of the foetus make this choice freely.

or leads to more irreconcilable family conflicts, that may be a problem in countries where the family is the primary social safety net for the indigent and old.[16]

But the main problem in promoting respect for autonomy in its standard bioethical guise is the effect of the standard analysis of the legitimacy of transactions, i.e. if a transaction is mutually beneficial and freely consented to it cannot be morally wrong and it should not be the object of legal interference.

Let us first note that there is no simple argument from 'not morally wrong' to 'no legal interference'. A significant amount of regulation of commercial transactions is aimed at increasing the societal efficiency of transactions and not at protecting either of the parties.

More importantly, however, a predictable side-effect of implementing the standard autonomy-based view, in a situation of significant persistent inequalities in bargaining power and resources, is that those with significant resources can serially exploit a series of mutually-beneficial exchanges to increase these inequalities. The feudal transactions between landlords and tenants were often of precisely this kind (as long as epidemics or wars did not deplete the supply of tenants and raise their 'price').

A cynical, but publicity-conscious pharmaceutical firm might for instance devise a well-calibrated benefit-sharing policy that at the same time ensures that enough benefit is shared so that the firm can claim that its research transactions are mutually beneficial, and so little benefit shared that the pool of research participants will never be in a position to realistically refuse future participation. And an astute organ brokerage firm will be able to exploit the vulnerabilities of both the parties to the transactions it brokers, while being able to claim the moral high ground of helping them to conclude a mutually-beneficial transaction.

What has gone wrong here is not the mere global promotion of respect for autonomy, but the promotion of one specific analysis of the morality of transactions which, in a situation with limited background injustice (or inequality for those who do not think that these inequalities are unjust) is relatively unproblematic, but which in a situation with huge background injustice has very significant negative side-effects. This problem can be rectified in different ways, either by being more sensitive to the importance of context, or by promoting justice with the same vigour as we promote autonomy. Or perhaps more accurately, promoting justice to such an extent that the requirements of justice have the same chance of being fulfilled as the requirements of respect for autonomy at the global level, or are fulfilled to the same degree. I will leave it to the reader to contemplate how that balance can be achieved given the rather dismal record of attempts to promote global justice.

16 In passing we may note that too vigorous a promotion of personal autonomy might actually contravene the literal meaning of Article 16.3 of the *Universal Declaration*.

Chapter 7
Health in Developing Countries and Our Global Responsibilities

Gillian Brock
University of Auckland, New Zealand

Do we have obligations to improve the health of those living in developing countries? It is often thought that there are no morally salient connections between us in developed countries and those in the developing world which would mean that obligations of justice are at issue here. Rather, at best, if we have any responsibilities towards improving the health of those in developing countries these are matters of charity or benevolence.

In this paper I argue that there are, indeed, some morally salient connections between 'us' and 'them' which mean that the responsibilities at issue are ones of justice. I discuss our international healthcare worker recruitment practices and the devastating effects these typically have on the health of those in developing countries, especially those whose health is most at risk. By failing to reform our current arrangements we are failing in our negative duty not to uphold or contribute to injustice. Our failure to reform such arrangements implicates us in the continuation of poor health in developing countries. Far from it being an optional matter of charity whether or not we assist developing countries, there are central matters of justice at stake.

What Is the Problem?

'Brain drain' occurs when many skilled citizens from a particular country emigrate, thus draining the country of workers with high levels of training and leaving behind the less skilled (or unskilled). This phenomenon can have noticeable effects for the country they exit. One area in which brain drain is devastating is the healthcare sector. Brain drain among health professionals is particularly widespread and damaging for developing countries. These countries typically already have poor healthcare resources, so the loss of trained healthcare workers is felt even more greatly than it might be in places that are better resourced.

Indeed, in some cases, recruitment of healthcare workers from developing countries threatens the viability of the healthcare systems in those countries, especially in sub-Saharan Africa. Consider, for instance, how in Zambia, only

50 of the 600 doctors that have been trained in the country since independence have remained there.[1] Furthermore,

> … in Africa alone, where health needs and problems are greatest, around 23,000 qualified academic professionals emigrate annually. Information from South African medical schools suggests that a third to a half of its graduates emigrate to the developed world. The loss of nurses has been even more extreme—for example, more than 150,000 Filippino nurses and 18,000 Zimbabwean nurses work abroad. A recent report from the United Kingdom estimated that 31% of its doctors and 13% of its nurses are born overseas; in London the figures are 23% and 47% respectively. These reported figures are likely to be underestimates as many migrate unofficially.[2]

The costs to developing countries of such losses are enormous.[3] Indeed, it is clear that in sub-Saharan Africa basic healthcare delivery is significantly threatened by this phenomenon.[4] In particular, the recruitment of foreign nurses by developed countries 'has grown to such proportions that it is affecting the sustainability of entire health systems in some developing countries, depriving them of knowledge, skills and expertise—often at the expense of governments that have paid for the education of these nurses'.[5] In some cases, countries lose more nurses every year than they train, for instance, in 2001 Ghana lost 500 nurses, which is more than double the number of new nurses who graduated in that year.[6]

Recruiting health workers to rich countries can have varying effects on source countries, sometimes benefiting them through additional remittances, training and experience. In some cases such as the Philippines, the country trains more nurses than it needs in order to supply foreign markets. Those workers then remit funds back to their family so these migrant workers can be an important source of foreign

---

1 P. Bundred and C. Levitt, 'Medical migration: who are the real losers?', *Lancet*, 356 (2000): 245-6. Cited in *Rural and Remote Health* at http://rrh.deakin.edu.au

2 Tikki Pang, Mary Ann Lansang, Andy Haines, 'Brain drain and health professionals: A global problem needs global solutions', *British Medical Journal*, 324 (2002): 499-500. We see similar figures for the US. See, for instance, Amy Hagopian, Matthew J. Thompson, Meredith Fordyce, et al., 'The migration of physicians from sub-Saharan Africa to the United States of America: measures of the African brain drain', *Human Resources for Health*, 2/17 (2004).

3 Pang, Lansang and Haines, 'Brain drain and health professionals', p. 500.

4 J.Huddart and O. Picazo, 'The health sector human resource crisis in Africa' (Washington DC: Bureau for Africa, Office of Sustainable Development, United States Agency for International Development, 2003); and A. Ehman and P. Sullivan, 'South Africa appeals to Canada to stop recruiting its MDs', *CMAJ*, 164 (2001): 387-8.

5 'Position statement on recruitment and rights of foreign nurses', p. 1. Available at: http://www.aft.org (accessed April 2006).

6 Ibid.

revenue. But it is overwhelmingly the case that for the vast majority of developing countries, the net effect is currently extremely negative, as I discuss.[7]

It is claimed that the lack of healthcare workers in developing countries such as those in sub-Saharan Africa, 'is an emergency that demands urgent action. The impact of healthcare worker migration from developing to developed countries is a significant component in this crisis'.[8] Losses in sub-Saharan Africa are said to be so dramatic that, according to some theorists 'the haemorrhage of health professionals from African countries is easily the single most serious human resource problem facing health ministries today.'[9] While many countries have actual and projected shortages of health workers, the shortages in sub-Saharan Africa are greatest where one million health workers are needed to meet the Millennium Development Goals by 2015. For countries which already have severe shortages of healthcare workers (as measured by being below one health worker per 1,000 population) further loss of workers is most likely to result in loss of health services and significant loss of health in the countries' populations. Furthermore, 'billion dollar funds amassed to address overwhelming global health problems (such as HIV/AIDS) are constrained primarily by the lack of healthcare professionals.'[10]

Arguably, it is not the total number of healthcare professionals that exist in the world at large that is a problem, but rather their distribution. Consider how, for instance, while only 21 per cent of the world's population resides in Europe and North America, they command 45 per cent of the world's doctors and 61 per cent of its nurses. Africa, which contains 13 per cent of the world population, has only three per cent of its doctors and five per cent of its nurses. There 'are only 750,000 health workers in all of sub-Saharan Africa, a region that serves 682 million people and suffers from 25 per cent of the world's burden of disease'.[11] That is to say, 1.3 per cent of the world's healthcare workers provide services to 13.8 per cent of the world's population in a region suffering 25 per cent of the world's disease burden. It is estimated that 2.5 health workers per 1,000 of population is needed for basic healthcare delivery.[12] Europe enjoys 10.3 per thousand, while Africa on

---

[7] See, for instance, 'Position statement on recruitment and rights of foreign nurses', p. 2.

[8] See 'The healthcare skills drain—a call to action', p. 1. Available at: http://www.bma.org.uk/ap.nsf/Content/skillsdrain (accessed May 4 2006).

[9] 'The ethics of overseas recruitment for global health', p. 3. Available at: http://www.ukglobalhealth.org/Default.aspx?textID=141&cSectionID=6 They also refer to the work of D. Sanders, D. Dovlo, W. Meeus, et al., 'Public health in Africa', in R. Beaglehole (ed.), *Global Public Health: A New Era* (Oxford: Oxford University Press, 2003), pp. 135-55.

[10] 'The healthcare skills drain—a call to action', p. 1, a report by the British Medical Association. Available at: http://www.bma.org.uk/ap.nsf/Content/skillsdrain (accessed May 2006).

[11] 'Ethical restrictions on international recruitment', p. 1.

[12] 'Teething problems in Africa's healthcare', in *The African Executive*. Available at: http://www.africanexecutive.com/modules/magazine/articles.php?article=699&magazine=

average has 1.4 per thousand. The World Health Organization has a target for the doctor to population ratio of 1 per 1,000. In the 25 poorest countries, the doctor patient ratio is only 1 per 25,000. (Currently the doctor to patient ratio is 1 per 500 in wealthy countries).[13]

When rich countries recruit workers trained in poor countries without compensation, what is effectively happening is that poor countries are subsidizing the healthcare of citizens of affluent countries, while losing significant healthcare resources in the process.

Why do so many healthcare professionals want to leave? Medical professionals cite reasons such as poor remuneration, bad working conditions, lack of professional development or promotional opportunities, lack of security, and lack of funding as important factors in their decision. Developed countries often appear to offer better pay, working conditions, or career and training opportunities not available in developing countries.

Furthermore, there are the recruitment practices of healthcare organizations in the developed world, which encourage and facilitate migration of healthcare workers. These practices can vary considerably, but include fairly active practices, such as, within a country already facing critical shortages, aggressively targeting the entire workforce of a particular hospital or region via recruitment agents (and thus stripping entire communities of their healthcare personnel). Other active practices include having recruitment booths at conferences known to attract healthcare workers from developing countries, or placing recruitment adverts in professional news sources with a large developing country readership. Some recruitment agencies have not followed basic good faith contracting principles and have given misinformation about the job, conditions, or pay, or misled workers into accepting jobs that are incompatible with their skills and experience. When I talk about recruitment practices here I will bracket such concerns entirely. I will be arguing that even if agreements that follow basic rules of fair contracting are struck between an individual healthcare worker and a healthcare organization, significant issues of justice remain.

What Has Been Done About the Problem?

The main response so far has been to establish codes of practice for the international recruitment of healthcare professionals. One of the most significant of these was that drawn up by the Department of Health of the United Kingdom, originally drawn up in 2001 and revised in 2004. It is supposed to guide all recruitment into the National Health Service. Some of the main guiding principles contained in the document are outlined next. It is noted first of all that international recruitment is a

---

71 (accessed May 2006)

13 'The ethics of overseas recruitment for global health', p. 3. Available at:http://www.ukglobalhealth.org/Default.aspx?textID=141&cSectionID=6 (accessed May 2006).

legitimate strategy in developing an adequate healthcare workforce, and that there are benefits that accrue to the individuals recruited, such as advanced training. The key principle which seems to do much of the justificatory work is that healthcare professionals may only be targeted for recruitment from developing countries for which there are government-to-government agreements with the United Kingdom that explicitly permit recruitment activities. However, if individuals from those countries volunteer themselves by personal application (rather than through a recruitment agency) they may be considered for employment. Other principles ensure that healthcare professionals are competent to practice in the United Kingdom, are protected by relevant law, and have equal access to support and further education.

The Department of Health's *Code of Practice* is also supplemented with a document outlining the best practice benchmarks for international recruitment. Here again we see the same point emphasized, 'There is no active recruitment of healthcare professionals from those developing countries that are included on the Department of Health website'.[14] However in discussion of that principle it is fully allowable that healthcare organizations may consider unsolicited applications from an individual who lives in a developing country if a personal application is made not using a recruitment agency.

Another key benchmark identified is that international recruitment should be 'sensitive to local healthcare needs so that international recruitment from any country should not destabilize local healthcare provisions'.[15] But taking this benchmark seriously would mean that recruitment from many countries (whether by personal application or not) will simply have to be prohibited if some of the facts cited in the first section are taken seriously, especially those concerning the crisis in healthcare in sub-Saharan Africa.

Noticeably absent from the UK code is any talk about compensation when individuals are recruited from developing countries. Why one might think that talk of compensation is relevant, is because there are a number of costs that a departing individual imposes on the society she leaves, especially when her training was subsidized by that society. Such costs include training, loss of service and health to the home country, and loss of revenue from taxed wages.

We do see talk of compensation in other codes, such as the *Commonwealth Code of Practice for the International Recruitment of Health Workers*, which I discuss next. The code aims to be sensitive both to the needs of recipient countries, but also the migratory rights of individual health professionals. The code intends to discourage the targeted recruitment of healthcare workers from countries that

---

[14] UK Department of Health of the United Kingdom,'Code of Practice for the international recruitment of healthcare professionals', p. 10, available at: http://www.dh.gov.uk/PublicationsAndStatistics/Publications/PublicationsPolicyandGuidance/PublicationsPolicyandGuidanceArticle/fs/en?CONTENT_ID=4097730&chk=D1/b1A (accessed May 2006).

[15] Ibid.

are already in dire situations with respect to healthcare. The key guiding principles are said to be 'transparency, fairness and mutuality of benefits as these relate to relations among Commonwealth countries, and between recruits and recruiters'.[16] Transparency usually requires that there is an agreement between the recruiting and source countries. Fairness requires a range of interesting responsibilities. For instance,

> The Code seeks to encourage the establishment of a framework of responsibilities between governments—and the agencies accountable to them—and the recruits. This framework would balance the responsibilities of health workers to the countries in which they were trained—whether of a legal kind, such as fulfilling contractual obligations, or of a moral kind, such as providing service to the country which had provided their training opportunities—and the right of health professionals to seek employment in other countries.[17]

Under mutuality of benefits we see encouragement for recruiters to 'consider ways in which they could provide assistance to source countries'[18] and that this could take the form of technical assistance, for instance.

The most interesting section is that subtitled 'Compensation/Reparation/ Restitution' which states that:

> Governments recruiting from other Commonwealth countries should/[may wish to] consider how to reciprocate for the advantages gained by doing so. This could include:
>
> - programmes to reciprocate for the recruitment of a country's health workers through the transfer of technology, skills and technical and financial assistance to the country concerned;
> - training programmes to enable those who return to do so with enriched value;
> - arrangements to facilitate the return of recruitees (subject to application of the non-discrimination principle and to the rights of the workers concerned in accordance with immigration and other laws).[19]

According to the code, governments should encourage good practice among recruitment agencies by dealing only with those that comply with the terms of the code. They should also monitor the practices of recruitment agencies. The code also specifies interesting views about workforce planning, such as, Principle 40 which states that: 'Where governments have expended resources to train, they may wish

16 'Commonwealth Code of Practice for the International Recruitment of Health Workers', p. 2. Available at: http://www.spnf.org.au/bulletin/codeofpractice.html (accessed May 2006).

17 Ibid., p. 2.

18 Ibid., p. 2.

19 Ibid., p. 3.

to consider strategies for ensuring that health professionals serve compulsorily for a specified period'.[20] Principle 41 encourages all countries to implement measures to retain skilled health workers, and to plan better for their workforce needs. This requires trying to improve the work environment through, for instance, improving conditions of service, opportunities for training, career development, and better pay. Strategies which some countries have used to decrease the international recruitment of health workers include: requiring compensation to be paid from departing workers trained at governments' expense, instituting compulsory service, increasing salaries, and improving benefits to healthcare workers (such as, education for children, transportation, housing or day care).

The desirability of non-commonwealth countries adopting the code is also mentioned (since, after all, we are in a global labour market). It is noted that international agencies, such as the World Health Organization (WHO), the World Medical Association, and the United Nations Educational, Scientific and Cultural Organization (UNESCO) could all play a role in trying to achieve respect for an international code.

Recently a code was adopted that, in theory at least, has global scope. This is the code entitled *Ethical Restrictions on International Recruitment of Health Professionals from Low-Income Countries* which was adopted at the World Federation of Public Health Associations.[21] The code specifies that healthcare workers are not to be recruited from developing countries unless there are government-to-government agreements, but even where there are such agreements,

> healthcare facilities incorporating workers from abroad are strongly encouraged to manage recruitment and incorporation of health care workers from those countries in such a way that the sending country receives something in return. Reciprocal strategies of this nature could include sending developed country health workers in an exchange program, remunerating the source government for its investment in a workers' education program, or offering continuing education that a foreign health worker could apply in the home country.[22]

Two other principles are noteworthy. First, Principle 6 which states that: 'Destination countries shall develop coordinated and comprehensive plans for monitoring the movement of physicians across their borders, and shall contribute to a fund at the World Health Organization that can assist sending countries to develop

---

20 Ibid., p. 6.

21 Several items are the same as other codes. For instance, though active recruitment is prohibited, employers are permitted to recruit individuals from developing countries if they receive unsolicited applications.

22 'Principle 1', p. 2. Available at: http://www.apha.org/private/2005_proposed_policies/D3_2005.pdf (accessed May 2006).

information systems to track the movement of their own health professionals'.[23] Second, according to Principle 9, destination countries need to commit to providing 'an adequate supply of human resources for health within their own borders and ensure appropriate workforce distribution, in order to discourage market-driven demand for health workers from abroad'.[24]

What Should be Done About the Problem?

So far, the codes have failed in numerous ways to solve the problem. First, the current codes are all voluntary. They simply specify the expectations one might have. But there are no real requirements for them to be followed. Recent research suggests that there are widespread violations of the UK code. Between March 2001 and 2002, twice the number of nurses were registered in the United Kingdom from South Africa as the year before in which there were no ethical recruitment guidelines.[25] In 2002-3, 'one in four new nurse registrants were from the "proscribed" list of countries—those listed in the Department of Health's *Code of Conduct* on international recruitment as not to be targeted by the UK's National Health Service (NHS) for active recruitment'.[26]

A major limitation of the UK code is that it only covers the NHS, and does not cover the independent or private sector. Furthermore, once someone has been employed by the private sector it becomes easier to move across to the NHS (as their immigration status may well have changed).

Codes alone will certainly not solve the recruitment problem. However, they do show some level of concern, set up some expectations for institutions aspiring to follow international benchmarks of good practice and, probably, the codes have slowed the rate of recruitment.

While having a voluntary code in place is a first step that can be taken, it is not a sufficient response. Governments can do much more than they are currently doing. Indeed, given that governments are the ones who supply visas to the potential recruits, it seems they have an excellent intervention point to do much more. When a potential recruit's visa is being considered, governments could make judgments on the projected impact of the recruitment, given what they do know about the source country, for instance, how many other visas have been granted to compatriots. Given this information, they could also sensibly recommend appropriate compensation for the home country (if the data warrants). This kind

---

23 Ibid., p. 3.

24 Ibid.

25 'The ethics of overseas recruitment for global health', p. 4. Available at: http://www.ukglobalhealth.org/Default.aspx?textID=141&cSectionID=6 (accessed May 2006).

26 Daloni Carlisle, 'UK's "ethical recruitment policy" needs to be strengthened', *British Medical Journal*, 328 (2004): 1218.

of scrutiny should apply whether the application is made through a recruitment agency—and so is considered active recruitment, or not.

However, what would really address the root of the problem more effectively is each country's achieving self-sufficiency with respect to healthcare resources. For developing countries, especially in sub-Saharan Africa, this means training more healthcare professionals. More resources need to be spent on investing in healthcare professionals. Where are the additional resources to come from? Some might certainly come from compensation for healthcare professionals poached from the developing world, but there are many other neglected sources. Helping developing countries themselves collect more of the revenue they are actually owed would be a major contribution. Elsewhere I show how reform to our international taxation arrangements (which are needed anyway on independent grounds) would make vastly greater sums of money available to developing countries.[27]

So, a comprehensive solution requires at least the following components: (1) an international code that specifies uniform standards for both private and public sectors, and which applies to all countries; (2) an international agency that oversees activities, brokers compensation, can punish violators (perhaps by levying fines) and so forth; (3) each country's aiming at and achieving self-sufficiency with respect to human resources in healthcare, and perhaps (4) addressing the seemingly insatiable demand for healthcare in developed countries.

Why Should Governments Take a More Active Role?

A full *positive* answer to this question requires me to say a whole lot more about our obligations of global justice to one another. This is a project undertaken elsewhere, that I do not have space to address here.[28] A very brief *positive* answer to this question might go like this: global justice requires that we are all adequately positioned to enjoy prospects for a decent life (that, in my view, is roughly fleshed out by what is necessary to be enabled to meet our basic needs and those of our dependents, and certain guarantees about basic freedom). Having adequate healthcare resources is a key part of that positioning. We all have responsibilities to one another to ensure social and political arrangements are in place to support central ingredients for a decent life. As agents who can act effectively on our behalf, governments can frequently help us to discharge our responsibilities. Protecting people's prospects for decent lives by ensuring they are adequately resourced with healthcare workers is one such significant occasion.

However, I do not have to give a complete, or indeed, any account of our *positive* obligations to one another to motivate the case that we have obligations to those in developing countries to attend to their healthcare crises in general and

[27] *Nationalism, Cosmopolitanism, and Global Justice* (Cambridge: Cambridge University Press, forthcoming), Chapter 5.

[28] Ibid., Chapter 3.

their lack of trained staff in particular. There are two pretty uncontroversial ways to argue this case.

First, via duties of compensation for past harms. In many cases the critical healthcare shortages they now face are a result of past active recruitment of healthcare workers that looks surprisingly like raiding other countries of their precious (human) resources. Our past actions on this front alone give rise to duties of rectification now. Minimally, those duties require a more active role, for instance, in monitoring the effects we are having on developing countries by recruiting their most skilled health workers, and either refusing visas to potential recruits who would exacerbate those problems or demanding that in exchange for the issuing of the relevant visa, the healthcare organization that would be employing the recruit offer adequate compensation to the source country.[29] Governments, as our agents of justice, must therefore play a more active role in, at the very least, ensuring we do not worsen the situation (though perhaps they also have responsibilities to offer more substantial compensation for the harm already perpetrated as well). So, according to this viewpoint, there are indeed some morally-salient connections between 'us' in developed countries and 'them' in developing ones—the way in which we have already taken resources from those who are most vulnerable is an important case of one such connection.

A second kind of argument can be marshaled via the negative duty we all have not to uphold or contribute to (current) injustice.[30] In taking such a casual approach to worsening the already dire situation of the global worst-off with respect to their healthcare (as I demonstrated in the first section), arguably we are failing to discharge this negative duty appropriately. By allowing the status quo to continue we are, in effect, failing in our negative duty to refrain from upholding unjust arrangements. To discharge this negative duty adequately, we need to make a more concerted effort, for instance, by having in place mandatory standards governing recruitment to ensure the situation does actually change to one more favourable to the world's most vulnerable people.

Would we be interfering unjustly with individuals' relevant freedoms, such as the freedom of movement or occupational freedom by, say, denying visas to individuals who were trained in countries with dire healthcare resources, who want to immigrate? I do not *necessarily* think so. The rights to emigrate that healthcare workers have must be balanced with the responsibilities those workers have to the countries in which they were initially trained. Perhaps if we denied these persons visas *unconditionally* we do interfere inappropriately. However, if we allow visas to be granted *on condition that the healthcare organization that would employ*

29 Of course, if we are going to recommend sound policy, we do need to gather as many facts as possible. Here I give an indication of the kind of policy that should be recommended given what we currently know about the situation. As more information is gathered, other policies might emerge as better ones.

30 See, for instance, Thomas Pogge, 'Priorities of global justice', *Metaphilosophy*, 32 (2001): 6-24.

them offer adequate compensation to the country of origin, this strategy strikes a reasonable balance, in my view.

In the first instance, it would be the departing individuals who would be responsible for paying compensation. But I assume that in many cases, probably the vast majority, making individuals solely responsible would effectively undermine their freedom of movement significantly, given their inability to pay compensation of the order of magnitude required. It is not unfair if the healthcare organizations that are employing emigrants and thereby deriving significant benefits from their employment should be made to absorb the costs. This proposal balances concern for individuals and the countries they depart more appropriately than other alternatives.[31]

[31] I am very grateful for the advice and suggestions made by Amy Hagopian in preparing this paper. For comments on an earlier draft, I am also very grateful to David Benatar and Martin Wilkinson.

Chapter 8
Shared Responsibility Agreements: Causes of Contention

Paula Boddington
Oxford University, UK

Introduction: Responsibility for Health and Shared Responsibility Agreements

Discussions about responsibility for health raise a great many complex issues, which are often obscured in the careless use of the term. Debates about the relative responsibilities of governments, individuals and communities for health need to occur against a background of clear thinking about the complex notion of responsibility. This chapter examines how claims about responsibility cohere with causal understandings of the health issues to be addressed.

Claims of responsibility for health are often made obliquely or by implication; here I discuss an example of overt claims about sharing responsibility for addressing various problems in Australian Aboriginal communities. My focus here is on the severe health problems of Indigenous Australians. Using measures such as life expectancy, which lags behind the population average by almost two decades, Aboriginal Australians' health is by far the worst of all comparable indigenous populations, and, moreover, has failed to make the improvements seen in other indigenous groups.[1]

The liberal Australian Government led by John Howard introduced in 2004 what is presented as a new arrangement in indigenous affairs, including Shared Responsibility Agreements (SRAs) with Aboriginal communities or other groups. These relate to a broad range of possible interventions, not simply those relating to health. However, the complex nature of the very serious health problems facing Indigenous Australians, which are quite clearly related to social and economic disadvantage, means that many SRAs, if not all, have some implication for health.

The Australian Federal Government explains Shared Responsibility Agreements thus:

---

[1] Ian Ring and Ngiare Brown, 'The Health Status of Indigenous Peoples and Others', *British Medical Journal*, 327 (2003): 404-5.

> An SRA is an agreement between government and community or some other kind of grouping, like a family or clan. It is focused on getting better results for indigenous people and sets out what all partners will do differently to make this happen … SRAs are about partnership. The Government wants communities to take responsibility for deciding on their own priorities for change and to work out what they can contribute to make things better.[2]

A community can set its own objectives and suggest an SRA to help meet these.[3] SRAs are not legally binding agreements enforceable by law.[4] The mechanism of accountability appears to lie in the principle of 'good faith', with no penalties for non-compliance, other than any political pressure that the government might find itself under for failure to keep its agreements.[5] If a community's agreements are broken the Government will consider not making any more with that community.[6] It is claimed that SRAs deal with the provision of discretionary benefits rather than basic services or entitlements and therefore do not infringe citizenship rights, and hence by implication are not discriminatory.[7]

There are many diverse examples of SRAs, concerning projects such as assistance with the provision of kidney dialysis support centres, the development of walking trails to preserve community history and stories, improvements to a water supply where this had been contaminated by feral animals, the provision of distance education, the provision of swimming pools, often linked to school attendance under 'no school, no pool' rules, the provision of community stores, for example after one at the Minjilang community in Arnhem Land was destroyed by a cyclone. In exchange, communities have undertaken various measures, including prompt payment of rents, rubbish removal, upkeep of pools and recreational

---

2 Australian Government, Office of Indigenous Policy Coordination, 'Australian Government Feature. Indigenous Affairs: Sharing Responsibility. Shared Responsibility Agreements Questions and Answers' Available at: http://www.indigenous.gov.au/rpa/koori_mail_ins.pdf (accessed April 2009).

3 Australian Government, Office of Indigenous Policy Coordination, 'Australian Government Feature. Indigenous Affairs: Sharing Responsibility. Shared Responsibility Agreements Questions and Answers'.

4 Kari M. S. Kristiansen and Kerriane Cox, 'Shared Responsibility Agreements: Legally or Morally Binding?', *Indigenous Law Bulletin*, 6/11 (2005): 8-11.

5 Amanda Vanstone, ABC Radio, 'Senator Amanda Vanstone' *Speaking Out*, 20 March 2005. Available at: http://www.abc.net.au/message/radio/speaking/stories/s1324685.htm (accessed April 2009).

6 Ruth McCausland, 'So Just Who is Sharing the Responsibility in Indigenous Policy?', *New Matilda*, 9 March 2005.

7 Vanstone, 'Senator Amanda Vanstone' *Speaking Out:* 'SRAs are not about imposing new conditions on the provision of citizen entitlements or essential services. They don't affect Centrelink benefits'.

facilities, and behaviours such as 'keeping store area tidy' and 'not pressuring the store staff for credit'.[8]

What Thinking Lies Behind Shared Responsibility Agreements?

The Australian Government has presented the introduction of SRAs in terms of a prevailing philosophy of equal opportunities.[9] An explicit aim is to foster and accept responsibility; claims are made that this should be a dual attempt by government and by communities.[10] It is important to realize that the situation is portrayed not simply as one of social and economic and health disadvantage. Additionally and importantly, an explicit aim is to overcome 'welfare passivity', seen by the government, controversially, as a problem generally and with Indigenous Australians in particular. This can be constructed as failure to take on board adequate responsibility.[11]

The Howard Government has espoused a philosophy of 'mutual obligation' underlying its welfare programmes, allegedly based upon the idea of a social contract and upon the idea that rights are accompanied by corresponding duties and obligations.[12] This underlying philosophical approach is applied generally, and also specifically to indigenous policy, where a shift from a policy based upon indigenous self-determination to one of mutual obligation can be seen to be taking place.[13] There has been a move away from a 'rights-based' agenda in indigenous

---

8 Information on SRAs in general and for individual SRAs can be found on the Australian Government's SRAs and RPAs website, http://www.indigenous.gov.au/sra.html#sra (accessed April 2009).

9 Senator the Hon. Amanda Vanstone, Minister for Immigration and Multicultural and Indigenous Affairs, message from Australian Government Feature: 'We wanted to do things differently because we know that indigenous people have not been getting a fair share of the opportunities Australia provides'. Available at: : http://www.indigenous.gov.au/rpa/common_ground.pdf (accessed April 2009).

10 Vanstone, 'Australian Government Changes to Indigenous Affairs Services Commence Tomorrow', Press releases, 30 June 2004. Available at http://www.atsia.gov.au/Media/former_minister/media04/v04039.aspx (accessed October 2006).

11 See 'The Howard Government Election 2004 Policy, Indigenous Australians: Opportunity and Responsibility'. Available at: http://www.nit.com.au/downloads/files/Download_53.pdf (accessed April 2009).

12 Pamela Kinnear, *Mutual Obligation: Ethical and Social Implications: Discussion paper number 32* (The Australia Institute, 2000).

13 See e.g. Ruth McCausland, 'Briefing Paper No. 1: Shared Responsibility Agreements' (Ngiya Institute for Indigenous Law, Policy and Practice, 2005). Available at: http://www.jumbunna.uts.edu.au/research/shared_responsibility.pdf. See also Jane Robbins, 'Life After ATSIC: Indigenous Citizenship in an Era of Mutual Obligation', (2005). Available at http://auspsa.anu.edu.au/proceedings/publications/Robbinspaper.pdf (both accessed April 2009).

affairs to one based upon what is termed 'practical reconciliation', allegedly focused upon achieving concrete results, and eschewing calls for what might be seen to be more symbolic calls for reconciliation.[14]

The mutual obligation philosophy has widespread acceptance, but its philosophical basis, as well as practical implications, have also attracted much criticism.[15] It has been pointed out that 'welfare dependency' is not clearly defined,[16] although it appears to refer to those who lack the will, rather than the capacity, for self-reliance.[17]

Indeed, some prominent Aboriginal leaders have spoken in terms that seem to align with what is called the 'war on welfare dependency':

> A number of Aboriginal leaders, ourselves included, have decided to combine our energies to advance the system of Aboriginal people from an abysmal state of social and economic inertia to a circumstance more closely approaching the reality of non-Aboriginal Australians.[18]

Dodson and Pearson talk of the 'failures of expectation' that lead to failures to take responsibility. However, caution is also voiced, warning for example that SRAs can be used to gain a leverage of control over the lives of Aboriginal people.[19]

The situations to be addressed are highly complex. SRAs are explicitly designed to be simple.[20] However, even if this may have pragmatic justification in certain cases, it can in some instances be a source of significant problems regarding attribution of responsibility where salient causal complexities are obscured. This will be explored in this paper, using an example of an SRA dealing with trachoma control. Many issues concerning the responsibility of different parties merit discussion: here the focus will be on the dangers of over-simplifying

---

14 K. Collard, H.A. D'Antoine, D.G. Eggington, B.R. Henry, C.A. Martin, G.H. Mooney '"Mutual" Obligation in Indigenous Health: Can Shared Responsibility Agreements be Truly Mutual?', *Medical Journal of Australia* 182/10 (2005): 503.

15 Kinnear, 'Mutual Obligation: Ethical and Social Implications'.

16 S. Parker, 'Welfare Dependency and the Logic of Mutual Obligation', *Just Policy*, 32 (2004): 28-35.

17 Ian Anderson, 'Mutual Obligation, Shared Responsibility Agreements and Indigenous Health Strategy', *Australia and New Zealand Health Policy*, 3 (2006): 10.

18 Pat Dodson, Noel Pearson, 'The Dangers of Mutual Obligation', *The Age* (Melbourne, 15 December 2004. Available at: http://www.theage.com.au/news/Opinions/The-dangers-of-mutual-obligation/2004/12/14/1102787075763.html (accessed April 2009).

19 McCausland, 'Shared Responsibility Agreements'.

20 Australian Government, Office of Indigenous Policy Coordination, 'Shared Responsibility Agreements and Regional Partnership Agreements'. Available at: http://www.indigenous.gov.au/sra/kit/what_are.pdf (accessed April 2009).

a complex situation. Questions arise about how a poor health, social, cultural and economic situation came about, and how, and by whom, it can be most effectively addressed. Disentangling the relative roles of government, communities and individuals can be vexed. However, failure to address the causation of issues and the misrepresentation of complex issues can, as will be argued, act to create damaging confusion. This confusion may sometimes mean that attributions of responsibility are made unfairly, and may impede attempts to find an effective solution to entrenched and difficult problems.

Critiques of Shared Responsibility Agreements

There has been much criticism of SRAs. Individual SRAs vary a great deal and so criticism apt for one may not be apt for another. Their assessment is complex: benefits may be mixed in with problems; for example practical advantages may come along with the promotion of an underlying philosophy that is undesirable for various reasons. This paper will focus on problems; this does not mean that some SRAs may offer some benefit to some communities. Here I briefly review the main criticisms that have been levelled at SRAs, and some of the replies that have been produced.

An often voiced group of concerns about SRAs is that they are paternalistic, patronizing and coercive,[21] and a form of 'barter',[22] the introduction of blackmail to obtain basic services,[23] and a form of social engineering, which even if unavoidable, needs to be handled with great care.[24] It has been argued that restrictive choice sets and the lack of resources for achieving important ends other than the negotiation of SRAs may mean even apparently voluntary agreements are unfair.[25]

Government responses to such criticisms include a relative justification claiming that SRAs aim to counter a worse form of paternalism of prolonged, possibly intergenerational, over-reliance upon government assistance leading to dependence and a 'culture of victimhood'. A relationship of trust between government and communities is also used as a defence against charges of

---

[21] One of many to produce such a criticism is Kim Carr, Indigenous Affairs Spokesman for the Australian Labor Party. See M. Metherell, K. Gauntlett, 'Aborigines Strike Fuel for Hygiene Deal', *The Sydney Morning Herald* 9 December 2004.

[22] Anonymous, 'Practical Reconciliation or a New Level of Paternalism? Evaluating Shared Responsibility Agreements', *Just Comment*, Edmund Rice Centre for Justice and Community Education and The Australian Catholic University, 9/1 (2006).

[23] Metherell, Gauntlett. 'Aborigines Strike Fuel for Hygiene Deal'.

[24] Dodson, Pearson, 'The Dangers of Mutual Obligation'.

[25] McCausland, 'Shared Responsibility Agreements'.

paternalism.[26] Some Aboriginal commentators have also replied that Aboriginal people are fully capable of negotiating on their own terms with the government.[27]

Charges of discrimination are often made. It has often been claimed that, contrary to government statements, at least some SRAs impose conditions upon access to basic services that must be met by Indigenous Australians but not by others.[28] It has been said that 'mutual obligation' really means nothing more than placing conditions on the provision of indigenous funding.[29] There are serious concerns that SRAs represent an undermining of the integrity of a rights-based system, with serious questions of conditionality placed on indigenous people's citizenship entitlements.[30] It has been claimed that in making these judgements the special status of indigenous people must be taken into account. It also makes a significant difference who is expecting these behaviours: someone outside of the community, or an expectation generated internally to the community.[31] As we shall see, these issues relate strongly to the simplicity of SRAs and the way in which causally complex situations may be misrepresented.

Government response to the charge of discrimination claims that conditionality also applies to other Australians.[32] However this very conditionality, expressed in the 'mutual obligation' philosophy, has itself been argued to be an unfair distortion of rights that places burdens on those with least control over their lives, which would surely include Australia's indigenous population.[33]

In some instances, there seems to be no apparent connection between what the government is agreeing to provide and what the community has to do in return; this has been said to render such SRAs patronizing. The principle of mutual obligation has been said to be 'bastardized' when agreements have no 'logical and balanced

---

[26] Peter Shergold 'Government and Communities in Partnership: Sharing Responsibility', Speech, May 18 2005, http://www.pmc.gov.au/speeches/shergold/sharing_responsibility_2005-05-18.cfm (accessed October 2006).

[27] McCausland 'Shared Responsibility Agreements'.

[28] Metherell, Gauntlett. 'Aborigines Strike Fuel for Hygiene Deal'.

[29] ANTAR (Australians for Native Title and Reconciliation) Factsheet, 'Mutual Obligation, Shared Responsibility and Mainstreaming in Indigenous Affairs' .Available at: http://www.antar.org.au/index.php?option=com_content&task=view&id=95&Itemid=105, (accessed October 2006).

[30] Aboriginal Lawyer Michael Mansell has argued that placing funding conditions on agreements with indigenous communities mean these SRAs violate the Race Discrimination Act. Steve Pennels, 'Rules Unfair, Say Proud Mulan People', *The Age* (10 December 2004).

[31] Emma Kowal, 'Mutual Obligation and Indigenous Health: Thinking Through Incentives and Obligations', *Medical Journal of Australia*, 184/6 (2006): 292-3.

[32] Shergold, 'Government and Communities in Partnership: Sharing Responsibility'; for example, the requirement actively to look for work whilst in receipt of unemployment benefits.

[33] Kinnear, 'Mutual Obligation: Ethical and Social Implications'.

set of rights and responsibilities'.[34] The situation may seem coercive or patronizing especially if there are power imbalances, as would typically be seen between a government and a small community, and if the legitimacy of the exercise of power is called into question.[35] Furthermore, without adequate alternatives, and the more basic the services the community wishes for, the stronger the element of coercion.[36] The thought that indigenous people are being treated like naughty children underlies the warning of Aboriginal Democrat Senator, Aden Ridgeway, that SRAs have the 'potential to turn into blackmail with the Government withholding essential resources until communities fall into line—what we have heard are simplistic slogans of "no school, no pool", "no wash, no money". What will be next, "no greens, no dessert"? Does anyone really believe this will work?'.[37]

The Simple, 'Results-Oriented' Nature of SRAs

Many criticisms of SRAs have cited their simplicity. It is claimed that the complex nature of indigenous disadvantage may become oversimplified.[38] They are criticized for being *ad hoc*. SRAs are by their very nature conducted at the micro level, and do not relate to systematic, and therefore possibly much more effective, policy.

They are also simplistic in that they are explicitly going for *results* only. There is no basis in any underlying recognition of how the current situation of Indigenous Australians arose. Thus, as well as the empirical question of whether such a simple approach can work, this very simplicity additionally raises normative issues.

It is instructive to consider this focus on concrete results rather than on the symbolism of apology in the context of the very broadly holistic Aboriginal definition of health, which includes not only physical, social and emotional well-being, but also the 'cultural well-being of the whole community'.[39] Many take the

---

[34] Kristiansen and Cox, 'Shared Responsibility Agreements: Legally or Morally Binding?'.

[35] Many point to the power imbalances as an underlying reason to consider an element of paternalism in the agreements. See e.g. McCausland, 'So Just Who is Sharing the Responsibility in Indigenous Policy?'.

[36] Dodson, Pearson, 'The Dangers of Mutual Obligation'.

[37] Metherell, Gauntlett, 'Aborigines Strike Fuel for Hygiene Deal'.

[38] Kristiansen and Cox, 'Shared Responsibility Agreements: Legally or Morally Binding?'.

[39] 'Aboriginal health is not just the physical well being of an individual but is the social, emotional and cultural well being of the whole community in which each individual is able to achieve their full potential thereby bringing about the total well being of their community. It is a whole-of-life view and includes the cyclical concept of life-death-life. Health to Aboriginal peoples is a matter of determining all aspects of their life, including control over their physical environment, of dignity, of community self-esteem, and of justice. It is not merely a matter of the provision of doctors, hospitals, medicines or the

view that symbolic acts, such as an apology from the government for past abuses, is causally necessary to address health and other issues.[40] [41]

Underlying notions of how the current problems of Indigenous Australians have arisen are surely relevant to an adequate causal understanding of their situation. From one understanding, an approach may be seen to be *simple yet effective* if it 'goes to the heart of the matter', and simplicity may be a virtue cutting through irrelevance or unmanageable complexity; from another understanding, what is simple may be seen to be merely 'simplistic'.[42]

Aboriginal commentators take different positions on the causation of current problems. Noel Pearson, based on his experience in Cape York, considers that the provision of welfare is itself a direct cause of Aboriginal passivity.[43] Others dispute this analysis, focusing instead upon the complex web of social, cultural, and economic factors that have impacted upon Indigenous Australians since European settlement, including dispossession and the forced removal of children.[44] Whatever view is taken, some analysis of what has created a situation of disadvantage is necessary to address the question of whether SRAs are equitable. Examining the mutual obligation philosophy in relation to unemployment benefits, Kinnear has forcefully argued that an analysis of the root cause of systemic unemployment shows the inequity of placing conditions on benefits and on construing individual behaviour as the cause of unemployment.[45]

---

absence of disease and incapacity'. National Aboriginal Strategy Working Party, *A National Aboriginal Health Strategy* (Canberra, Department of Aboriginal Affairs, 1989). This is a very well accepted and widely-used definition.

40 For example, it has been argued that reconciliation is causally necessary to address health problems, drawing upon comparisons with other countries such as Aotearao/NZ where a formal treaty exists. Lisa R. Jackson, Jeanette Ward, 'Aboriginal Health: Why is Reconciliation Necessary?', *Medical Journal of Australia* 170 (1999): 438.

41 Hermeston argues that a genuine 'true apology' for past injustice 'would go some way towards making holistic health gains and dealing with health inequities experienced by Aboriginal and Torres Strait Islander people'. Wendy A, Hermeston, 'Telling You Our Story: how Apology and Action Related to Health and Social Problems in Aboriginal and Torres Strait Islander Communities', *Medical Journal of Australia* 183/9 (2005): 438.

42 Aden Ridgeway has called them 'simplistic': dealing with behavioural issues will not counter poverty. Metherell Gauntlett, 'Aborigines Strike Fuel for Hygiene Deal'.

43 Noel Pearson, 'Positive and Negative Welfare and Australia's Indigenous Communities', *Family Matters*, 54 (1999): 30-35.

44 For a discussion of this see e.g. McCausland, 'Shared Responsibility Agreements'; Anderson, 'Mutual Obligation, Shared Responsibility Agreements and Indigenous Health Strategy'; see also Human Rights and Equal Opportunity Commission, 'Bringing Them Home: Report of the National Inquiry into the Separation of Aboriginal and Torres Strait Islander children From Their Families', (Sydney NSW: April 1997).

45 Kinnear, 'Mutual Obligation: Ethical and Social Implications'.

Likewise, an understanding of the reasons behind indigenous disadvantage is essential for assessing the equity of SRAs.

The Complex Nature of Responsibility

A glaring feature of the Australian SRA debate is that the word 'responsibility' is bandied about with little apparent awareness of different notions of responsibility. Responsibility, both causal and moral, can be attributed not just to individual agents but also to groups of people and institutions such as communities, governments and other agencies. A distinction needs to be made between causal responsibility for having created a situation and different types of moral responsibility for addressing it. Crucially too, attributions of moral responsibility may or may not carry with them judgements of culpability or blame. There is much that can be said on this matter. But a person, or group of people, may be said to have responsibility for addressing a situation because they have brought it about and are therefore possibly seen as culpable in some way; or they may have responsibility placed upon them, or take it on voluntarily, in a manner that in no way indicates any degree of culpability, or even causal involvement in creating the situation.[46] Although attributions of moral responsibility do not necessarily follow in any straightforward manner from an analysis of causal responsibility, nonetheless, a clear and accurate understanding of causation is an essential basis for clear thinking about responsibility.

An additional complication is that it cannot necessarily easily be said that there is one correct or complete causal analysis of any situation, and this is especially the case with the health problems that particularly impact upon the Australian Aboriginal population, which includes diseases recognized to have complex origins such as coronary artery disease and type 2 diabetes. Emphasis on different causes can have practical and ideological ramifications.[47]

Additionally, there are concerns about how responsibility can effectively and decently be cultivated in another, especially in a situation of unequal power, and against an historical background of colonization. Commentators suggest that encouragement from the outside can foster trust, respect and reciprocity but trying to enforce these on a community will not work and may be deleterious, and may violate international law.[48]

---

[46] There are many philosophical discussions of responsibility, see for example Jonathan Glover, *Responsibility* (London, Routledge and Kegan Paul: 1970).

[47] Ulla Räisänen, Marie-Jet Bekkers, Paula Boddington, Srikant Sarangi, Angus Clarke, 'The Causation of Disease: The Practical and Ethical Consequences of Competing Explanations', *Medicine Health Care and Philosophy*, 9/3 (2006): 293-306.

[48] 'The rationale is social control which breaches international obligations under Article 1 of the *International Covenant on Civil and Political Rights*, giving rights to self-determination'. K. Collard, H.A. D'Antoine, D.G. Eggington, B.R. Henry, C.A. Martin,

Essentially, an issue raised is the paradox of attempting to force people to become responsible. This issue is discussed in fairly explicit terms of internalization or externalization of behaviour by some of the commentators.[49] It also relates pragmatically to the goals of health (or other) policy. The question has been posed whether it is acceptable for people to change their behaviour in order to get a reward or whether this must be rooted in a genuine belief in the related health benefits. This is matter of both effectiveness and of ethics.[50] It has been sceptically asked whether government policy would expect white people to produce sustained behaviour change in response to external rewards.[51] The issues are somewhat different if community leaders are themselves encouraging behaviour change, but this then raises issues such as the nature of the leadership and possible internal community dissent and disagreement. As later discussion will show, causal understandings of a situation will impact upon understandings of who legitimately owes responsibility to whom.

The Mulan SRA: The 'Simple' Trading of Fuel for Health

SRAs vary considerably and hence it is important to consider the detail of individual agreements.[52] The first SRA with the Mulan people of Western Australia has attracted much discussion. Here it will be used to illustrate quite specific problems with causation and how this impacts upon understandings of responsibility: in this case, the causal origins of a specific disease are at issue.

The first Mulan SRA was a 'simple' formula with economic and health aims: the provision of petrol bowsers (pumps) in exchange for basic hygiene steps designed to lower the high rates of trachoma and other infestations amongst children.

G.H. Mooney, '"Mutual" Obligation in Indigenous Health: Can Shared Responsibility Agreements be Truly Mutual?', *Medical Journal of Australia* 182/10 (2005): 503.

49 Collard et al., '"Mutual" Obligation in Indigenous Health'.

50 Kowal, 'Mutual Obligation and Indigenous Health'.

51 Anderson, 'Mutual Obligation, Shared Responsibility Agreements and Indigenous Health Strategy'.

52 Many comment on the highly variable nature of SRAs, see e.g. ATSI (Aboriginal and Torres Strait Islander) Social Justice Commissioner 'Social Justice Report 2005 Factsheet 2: Shared Responsibility Agreements'. Available at: http://www.humanrights.gov.au/social_justice/sj_report/sjreport05/sjr_2005_factsheet2.html (accessed April 2009).

Table 8.1 The first Mulan (Western Australia) Shared Responsibility Agreement[53]

The Indigenous community would:	*In exchange, the Government would:*
• Ensure children shower daily and wash their faces twice a day. • Ensure rubbish bins are at every house and are emptied twice weekly, through the local work-for-the-dole scheme. • Undertake household pest control four times a year. • Ensure the rubbish tip is properly managed. • Act to prevent petrol sniffing. • Make sure children attend school, crèche and health clinic. • Keep homes and yards clean and put rubbish in bins immediately. • Pay rents to ensure the local council can afford pest control and repairs like plumbing. • Work with Community Consulting Agents to monitor extent to which commitments are met.	• Federal Government to provide $172,000* for a petrol bowser which would (allegedly) attract tourists and provide extra income. • Western Australia Government to organise health checks for children, especially for trachoma, skin infections and worms. • and monitor and review the adequacy of local health services to ensure any ongoing issues e.g. trachoma, secondary skin infections and worm infestations, are identified and addressed.

* The University of Melbourne's Agreements, Treaties and Settlements Database records the figure of $221,000. Available at: http://www.atns.net.au/biogs/A002622b.htm (accessed October 2006).

The previous petrol bowser had rusted out, making a 90km round trip to the nearest; the community had been asking for one for some time. Eventually after a reported 'tip off' from someone in government that an SRA might work, the community obtained this agreement.[54]

There has been much criticism of this particular SRA concerning both its formal structure and the practicalities of its inception and implementation. For example, it has been charged that as a business venture it manifestly lacked costings or any analysis of how it might impact on other communities.[55] It has also been claimed that not all community members were aware of or had agreed to the SRA.[56]

---

53 Available at: http://www.alp.org.au/download/mulan1204.pdf (accessed April 2009).

54 McCausland, 'Shared Responsibility Agreements: Practical Reconciliation or Paternalistic Rhetoric?'.

55 For example, Jon Altman quoted in Mark Coulton and Mark Metherell, 'A New Deal for Indigenous Australia', *Sydney Morning Herald*, 11 December 2004.

56 McCausland, 'So Just Who is Sharing the Responsibility in Indigenous Policy?'.

Moreover, although it has been widely reported that trachoma rates dropped as a direct result of the SRA,[57] it transpired that the community had themselves 18 months previously instigated a face-washing programme.[58] It has been widely claimed that as a result, trachoma rates had already dropped considerably before the implementation of the agreement,[59] but that government and other literature cited old statistics in justifying the agreement.[60] However, the situation is hard to assess as trachoma rates can fluctuate widely from season to season and the relevant statistics vary.[61]

Disease Causation and Responsibility

Media reports and government accounts stressed the high rates of trachoma in indigenous populations, especially in Mulan, comparing this unfavourably even to rates in the developing world.[62] 'Trachoma is an eye disease usually only found in the third world and the number one cause of preventable blindness in children ages 10-16'.[63] It looks like then a 'developing world disease', a disease of 'the other'. Which causes of a situation are highlighted will depend, *inter alia*, on what aspects of that situation stand out as most in need of explanation; this in turn can depend on context and on how a story is told.

The accompanying stress on face washing in this SRA means that an impression is easily gained that trachoma is, in essence, 'caused by' lack of hygiene.[64] In turn, these poor levels of hygiene in the young may be thought to be caused by failure on the part of adults to do something others would consider really basic; unfavourable attributions of responsibility, whether articulated or not, are not far off. Dodson and Pearson's claim that when actively engaged, taking responsibility

---

57 E.g. see Alan Mascarenhas, 'I Can See Clearly Now', *Sydney Morning Herald*, 12 May 2005.

58 McCausland, 'Shared Responsibility Agreements: Practical Reconciliation or Paternalistic Rhetoric?'.

59 See e.g. David Cooper, 'The Government's Much Heralded Shared Responsibility Agreements with Aboriginal Communities are Merely Window Dressing', *The Courier Mail*, 10 December 2005.

60 McCausland, 'So Just Who is Sharing the Responsibility in Indigenous Policy?'.

61 Anderson, 'Mutual Obligation, Shared Responsibility Agreements and Indigenous Health Strategy'.

62 Metherall, Gauntlett, 'Aborigines Strike Fuel for Hygiene Deal'.

63 Anonymous, 'Practical Reconciliation or a New Level of Paternalism?'.

64 For example, it is reported that 'Face washing is the simplest way to prevent trachoma'; a glib reading of this gives the impression that it is an easy and effective solution (Mascharenhas, 'I Can See Clearly Now'). However others stress that there are reasons to doubt this. Anderson, 'Mutual Obligation, Shared Responsibility Agreements and Indigenous Health Strategy'.

comes naturally out of 'natural love and regard for their own' and does not need to be engineered, also seems to underline the oddness of parents apparently failing to take basic care of their children.[65]

Trachoma becomes easily presented to the mainstream population as a disease that 'other people' get, as a result of scarcely explicable behaviour. But this presents a highly misleading picture.

Australia is the only developed country of the 57 trachoma endemic countries listed by the World Health Organization (WHO). However, the disease was endemic in many Western countries including Australia until about 1900, disappearing with improvements in socio-economic status, living conditions and hygiene. These improvements have not yet occurred in remote Aboriginal populations in Australia where trachoma is still endemic.[66]

Such an analysis immediately changes our perspective on trachoma, from something 'other' to Australia, to something that was once familiar and which the majority of the population has left behind. The 'cause' in the indigenous populations still affected by the disease then begins to look much more like the fact that they have not benefited equally from the social and economic advances to which the rest of Australia has been privy. In fact the causation of trachoma is extremely complex.[67]

As well as broad societal effects, explicit government action, or rather inaction, is implicated. Australia's trachoma-control efforts have been patchy since a national trachoma programme finished in 1978. Epidemiological data on trachoma are difficult to obtain and interpret because every programme has its own data recording system. Recent research shows that it is a highly mobile disease that could therefore benefit from enhanced inter-regional co-ordination.

The complexity of the disease process is revealed in national guidelines covering trachoma screening, control and data collection, and which stress the importance of implementing all four components of a SAFE strategy (surgery, antibiotics, facial cleanliness, environmental health). Responsibility for implementing the guidelines is specifically assigned to government-run regional population health units, working in collaboration with primary healthcare services and Aboriginal Community representatives.[68] Facial cleanliness is but one of these; moreover, it is actually unclear how effective face washing is in the control of the disease.[69]

---

65 Dodson, Pearson, 'The Dangers of Mutual Obligation'.

66 Donna B. Mak, 'Better Late than Never: a National Approach to Trachoma Control', *Medical Journal of Australia*, 184/10 (2006): 487-8.

67 Ibid.

68 Communicable Disease Network of Australia (CDNA), *Guidelines for the Public Health Management of Trachoma in Australia*; (Canberra, Australian Department of Health and Ageing, 2006); Mak, 'Better Late than Never: a National Approach to Trachoma Control'.

69 Anderson, 'Mutual Obligation, Shared Responsibility Agreements and Indigenous Health Strategy'.

The picture painted here is very far removed from the impression of disease causation and responsibility that it is easy to glean from the simplistic philosophy of the Mulan agreement and its official and unofficial discussion. It is said that 'they [the trachoma guidelines] provide yet more impetus for further and broader initiatives to address socio-economic deprivation, the underlying cause of continued trachoma transmission in Australian Aboriginal communities'.[70] Only a coordinated approach to trachoma control, rather than a patchwork of disparate deals, would be adequate.

Selective focus on certain causes of a disease can sometimes be pragmatically effective. Government responses to criticism of SRAs have typically made this point and describe SRAs as 'focused on getting better results for indigenous people ... If this agreement goes ahead, and it works, what could anyone complain about? A community gets what it wants, a petrol bowser. And the kids get better health outcomes'.[71] But the example of trachoma shows that if the focus is on results, national initiatives, not just local, are vital.

Moreover, focus on results may also obscure questions of the origin of the problems to be addressed; yet looking at origins may be essential to answer not just more practical questions, but questions about justice, equity, responsibility and entitlement. An agreement that made it look as if disease rates were down to the fecklessly irresponsible behaviour of parents creates a false impression. Moreover, an agreement that puts government in the position of cajoling these parents into accepting responsibility by the provision of an external reward reinforces the impression of lack of responsibility.

Questions of who has responsibility for various tasks or provisions depend amongst other things upon whether something is a right or an entitlement. Again, simplification of complex situations, together with the emphasis on 'results' as well as the lack of reference to the complex origins of indigenous disadvantage, means that questions about citizenship entitlements and rights for Indigenous Australians are again obfuscated, as many have remarked on in the context of mutual obligation.[72] In the arena of health alone, it has been argued that there is a growing body of evidence that Indigenous Australians do not receive the same level of medical care as others, an injustice linked to harmful ethnic stereotyping, from which it is concluded that 'the responsibility for reducing ethnic disparities

---

70 Mak, 'Better Late than Never: a National Approach to Trachoma Control': p. 488.

71 Australian Government, Office of Indigenous Policy Coordination, Australian Government Feature, 'Indigenous Affairs: Sharing Responsibility. Shared Responsibility Agreements Questions and Answers'. Available at: http://www.indigenous.gov.au/rpa/koori_mail_ins.pdf (accessed October 2006).

72 See e.g. Jane Robbins, 'Life After ATSIC: Indigenous Citizenship in an Era of Mutual Obligation', paper presented at APSA conference (Otago, September 2005). Available at: http://auspsa.anu.edu.au/proceedings/publications/Robbinspaper.pdf (accessed October 2006).

rests primarily with the healthcare system and its providers'.[73] There is a strong case to be made that the historical dispossession of Indigenous Australians, and the resulting loss of culture, community and family, are also causal factors in the high rates of illness and disease.[74] These considerations may well ground claims that indigenous people have strong entitlements to steps to decrease health disparities.

The simplicity of SRAs and their uncoordinated, *ad hoc* nature helps further obscure the causal origins of Aboriginal disadvantage; which in turn muddies the question of whether or not goods or services could decently be said to be 'privileges' or entitlements. If the latter, the conditionality attached to them can be strongly argued to be unjust.

Conclusions

When a government publication quotes the then Minister for Indigenous Affairs as saying 'as a result [of signing various SRAs] indigenous communities have been able to take responsibility for addressing issues they've identified through the SRAs'[75] the conflation of different aspects of responsibility is almost inevitable. Such mistaken attributions can happen regardless of the intention of governments, and are liable to be an unhelpful distraction from the important task of grappling with the complex issues of indigenous disadvantage.

It has been remarked that public perception of Indigenous Australians is a vital key to support for government policies. In fact, opinion polls show that Australians are divided on whether indigenous disadvantage represents continuing mistreatment or is the fault of indigenous people themselves.[76] Concern about public perceptions is expressed by many, including Dodson and Pearson: 'However, there is a risk that public opinion will place most of [the] blame for the present crisis on Aboriginal people'.[77] Many concerned about this Mulan SRA have pointed out that it shifts attention on indigenous behaviour as a problem requiring a solution, rather than on more systemic reasons such as policy failures.[78] The ways in which

---

73 Joan Cunningham, Alan Cass, Peter C. Arnold, 'Bridging the Treatment Gap for Indigenous Australians', *Medical Journal of Australia*, 182/10 (2005): 505-6.

74 Hermeston, 'Telling You Our story: How Apology and Action Related to Health and Social Problems in Aboriginal and Torres Strait Islander Communities'.

75 Senator Amanda Vanstone, 'Minister Announces 44 New SRAs with Indigenous Communities', VIPS 42/05. Available at: http://www.atsia.gov.au/media/former_minister/media05/v0543.aspx, (accessed October 2006).

76 Mark Burne, 'Reconciliation: Stalled, Fermenting, or Taken Out the Back and Shot?', *New Matilda*, 30 November 2005.

77 Dodson, Pearson, 'The Dangers of Mutual Obligation'.

78 See e.g. Antar (Australians for Native Title and Reconciliation) Factsheet, 'Shared Responsibility Agreements: A Critique'. Available at: http://www.antar.org.au/index.php?optoin=com_content&task=view&id=96&Itemid=105 (accessed October 2006).

this SRA has been hailed as a success for the Australian Government means that it conceals community initiative, misrepresenting the indigenous community.[79] Conversely, fears have been expressed that if SRAs are put in place that have scant chance of effective results, this could reinforce feelings of failure in Aboriginal communities.[80]

There may be good reasons to try to address questions of helplessness, hopelessness and inertia within Aboriginal communities. The fact that SRAs are intended to be practically based, simple, short term and do not necessarily have any logical connection between input and output, together with the use of the rhetoric of responsibility, means that they are a prime site for the mistaken attribution of responsibility and for continuing stereotyping and oversimplification of the complex and pressing issue of indigenous health.[81]

---

[79] Many have made this point; see e.g. Cooper, 'The Government's Much Heralded Shared Responsibility Agreements with Aboriginal Communities are Merely Window Dressing'.

[80] Anderson, 'Mutual Obligation, Shared Responsibility Agreements and Indigenous Health Strategy'.

[81] This work forms part of the project 'Explanations in Genetics: Causality and Accountability in Complex Disorders', funded by the Wellcome Trust and managed by Srikant Sarangi, Angus Clarke, Ruth Chadwick and Jenny Kitzinger, with research associates Marie-Jet Bekkers, Ulla Räisänen and Paula Boddington.

Chapter 9
Anti-Paternalism and Public Health Policy: The Case of Product Safety Legislation

Kalle Grill
Royal Institute of Technology, Stockholm, Sweden

The UK *General Product Safety Regulations 2005* state that products may not be brought to market if they present more than 'the minimum risk compatible with the product's use, considered to be acceptable and consistent with a high level of protection for the safety and health of persons'.[1] This recent regulation grants enforcement authorities the power to have products withdrawn from the market and recalled from buyers, and extended powers to halt the process of bringing a product to market.[2] In other words, decisions on acceptable risks from consumer products are to a considerable extent placed with government authorities, decisions that would otherwise be made by individual consumers. The UK regulation is based on a 2001 European Union directive; similar regulations apply throughout the Union, as well as in some other countries.

The risks involved in using consumer products are often risks to the user herself, rather than to third parties. Product safety regulation therefore typically involves paternalism. This article aims to distinguish the paternalistic content of product safety regulation, and in so doing, provide a more general framework for distinguishing the paternalistic content of any public health policy. Distinguishing the paternalistic content of policy is important if we want to evaluate the widespread resistance to paternalism codified in liberal anti-paternalist principles.

Most accounts of paternalism can be accommodated by the general definition *interference with a person, against her will, for her good*.[3] In the following, each of these three components will be discussed and applied to the case of product safety regulation, without commitment to a certain specification of any of the components. Concerning interference, I will consider five aspects of product safety regulation that make it an interfering policy, aspects that are relevant for public health policy more generally. Concerning will, I shall focus on the complexities arising from the fact that policies affect many persons and so can be welcomed or accepted for

[1] *The General Product Safety Regulations 2005*, Statutory Instruments 2005 no. 1803, p. 4.

[2] Peter Cartwright, 'Enforcement, risk and discretion: the case of dangerous consumer products', *Legal Studies*, 26/4 (2006): 524-43.

[3] Or an interference with several people against their will for their good.

quite different reasons. Concerning good, I will consider the important and often misunderstood role of reasons in understanding paternalism, again with special attention to many person cases. This three-fold interpretation will then be used to discuss the normative status of paternalism and anti-paternalism in public health policy. Throughout, references to the philosophical debate are largely confined to the footnotes.

Interference

For there to be paternalism, there must be some kind of interference on the part of the paternalist. Involvement with a person, merely affecting her in some way, is not enough. Interference may generally be thought of in terms of restriction or limitation of liberty. It is, however, a matter of controversy how the line should be drawn between innocuous involvement and interference. Disagreement may arise both concerning which concrete actions qualify as interference and concerning how interference should be specified in general terms. There are (at least) five reasons for holding that product safety regulation amounts to interference.[4]

First, regulation restricts options.[5] Less safe products may quite possibly have more or other functions and designs. Prohibiting the market exchange of less safe products thus restricts the options of individual consumers in a non-trivial sense. Importantly, the restriction of options may matter also for a person who would not have taken advantage of those options had they been available. Freedom is arguably about having more options available than those you actually choose to realize.[6]

Second, as a special case of restriction of options, regulation imposes a cost on the individual consumer. It is in general more expensive to produce safer products. If nothing else, the process of ensuring that the product is safe and that it accords

[4] I will assume throughout that those affected by the policy are sufficiently mature, informed, competent, and so on, to qualify as potential targets of illegitimate paternalism, according to liberal principles. The exact specification of these factors is an important and difficult matter for any anti-paternalist principle. The most ambitious attempt to accommodate this difficulty is arguably Joel Feinberg's in *Harm to Self* (Oxford: Oxford University Press, 1986), especially Chapter 20.

[5] Restriction of options has been taken to constitute interference by e.g. David Archard ['Paternalism defined', *Analysis* 50/1 (1990): 36] proposing as one condition of paternalism that a person 'P aims to bring it about that with respect to some state(s) of affairs which concerns [another person] Q's good Q's choice or opportunity to choose is denied or diminished'.

[6] Isaiah Berlin ['Five essays on liberty: introduction', in *Liberty* (Oxford: Oxford University Press, 2002 (1969)): 41] remarked that '[t]he extent of a man's negative freedom is, as it were, a function of what doors, and how many, are open to him; upon what prospects they open; and how open they are'. It is, of course, not obvious that the net effect of regulation will be a loss of liberty so understood.

with relevant regulation entails a cost. Consumers are in effect forced to spend money on safety features. If they were allowed to choose from a wider range of products, they should be able to find less expensive products that would serve the same purpose as more expensive, safer products. In the long run, the aggregated cost of safety may be quite high.

Third, because of the above traits of product safety regulation, it may go against the preferences of individual consumers.[7] People may value the opportunity to buy less safe products because they are less expensive, or because they have more or other functions, or simply because of a preference for simple, old-fashioned, or 'raw' products. People may also prefer to have options available that they do not in fact want to take advantage of.

Fourth, the purchase and use of consumer products is a typically private affair. Whether individuals use safe or less safe products usually has no direct effects on other people, or on society at large. There are of course indirect effects of people having accidents and subsequently becoming a burden on their loved ones and more generally on the healthcare system, while contributing less to society. Such effects may ensue, however, from all kinds of actions, however private. If there is such a thing as an area of personal sovereignty or a region of liberty, as anti-paternalists typically claim, the purchase of consumer products seems a good candidate for inclusion under this domain.[8]

Fifth, product safety regulation is backed up by criminal sanctions. It thus qualifies as interference also on those narrow accounts of paternalism that are restricted to the criminal law.[9] That the law punishes the seller rather than the buyer might make this a case of 'impure' paternalism, or a 'two party case'—the direct interference is with one party and the concern is with the health of the other party. On the other hand, since the buyer is an active and willing party to a mutual agreement, she too may be interfered with by the threat of sanctions to the seller.

---

[7] Donald Van de Veer [*Paternalistic Intervention* (Princeton: Princeton University Press, 1986): pp. 18-19] proposes that an action is an interference if the agent deliberately acts 'contrary to the operative preference, intention, or disposition of the subject' (or if she shapes or modifies these preferences in certain ways).

[8] Feinberg's (Chapter 19) account of paternalism rests heavily on the concept of personal sovereignty and the distinction between self-and other-regarding decisions; John Stuart Mill ['On liberty', in *On Liberty and Other Essays*, Oxford: Oxford University Press, 1991 (1859): p. 16] explains his anti-paternalist principle of liberty by pointing to 'the appropriate region of human liberty' as being 'that portion of a person's life and conduct which affects only himself, or if it also affects others, only with their free, voluntary, and undeceived consent and participation'.

[9] Feinberg explicitly restricts the domain of his anti-paternalist principle to criminal prohibition. There is a discrepancy between this narrow occupation with the criminal law and the fact that Feinberg's main argument against paternalism is based on the broad concept of personal sovereignty, see Richard Arneson, 'Joel Feinberg and the justification of hard anti-paternalism', *Legal Theory*, 11 (2005): 262-3.

Whether or not the interference is also with the buyer, these kinds of sanctions are typically and reasonably held to potentially involve paternalism.[10]

There are many ways to specify interference and every specification entails a different version of anti-paternalism. We may conclude, however, that there are several good reasons to count product safety regulation as interference. These reasons are quite general and may obviously apply also in other areas of public health policy. That product safety regulation is interfering does not of course mean that it is unjustified in all things considered, nor that it necessarily involves paternalism.

Will

That the effects of a policy goes against the preferences of a person subject to that policy is one reason to count the policy as an interference with that person, as noted above. However, preferences, or will, may also be considered an independent component of paternalism. If a policy constitutes an interference with a person on other grounds than going against her preferences, she may welcome the policy, fully aware of its interfering properties. We may want the government to ensure that there are no unsafe products available on the market, even if this restricts our options, because we do not think the risk of buying an unsafe product worth the possible benefits. The risks may include harm to oneself as well as the risk of harming others with the product (with possible liability). A policy that is welcomed on these grounds arguably does not involve paternalism. Importantly, it does not involve something that is opposed by liberal anti-paternalist principles.[11]

There are several choices to be made concerning the specification of the will component of paternalism. We may say that an interfering policy is unwelcome either when it goes against a person's expressed opinion, or when it is against her will or judgement, whether expressed or not, or whenever it does not have her expressed approval. We may also add conditions demanding that the approval or disapproval be more or less informed and competent.[12] Acknowledging that different interpretations of will lead to different versions of anti-paternalism, we may for our present purposes assume that a policy is normally welcomed by a person if she either explicitly approves of it, or would approve of it if the matter was brought to her attention.

As is now and then pointed out, public health policy differs from medical health contexts in that it affects large numbers of people, often in a non-discriminatory

---

[10] Gerald Dworkin, 'Paternalism', *Monist*, 56 (1972): 68; Feinberg, *Harm to Self*, p. 172.

[11] Mill ['On liberty' p. 14] typically opposes benevolent interference with a person only when it is 'against his will'.

[12] Again rising questions of what thresholds to accept, see fourth footnote in this chapter.

way.[13] This means that a policy may be welcomed for a number of different reasons. We should distinguish between welcoming the interfering effects of a policy on oneself, and accepting these effects as a necessary evil that is outweighed by the greater good of having the policy apply to all. The former case involves no more paternalism than an interference with one person that is welcomed by that person. Concerning the latter case, we should further distinguish between welcoming a policy because of the good effects for ourselves from interference with everybody else, and welcoming it because of the good effects on others from interference with them. As an example of the former, we may accept out of *self-interest* that the government ensures that we, as well as our neighbours, drive safely or keep our lawns tidy. As an example of the latter, we may accept out of *benevolence* that the government prevents us, as well as those more prone to addiction, from using heroin or tobacco. Similarly, we may accept interfering product safety regulation either because we do not want others to use dangerous products that may harm *us*, or we may accept it out of concern that they may harm *themselves*. A policy that interferes with us but that we welcome as a means to ensure compliance with a scheme that promotes our self-interest does, arguably, not involve paternalism for us.[14] On the other hand, it is undoubtedly paternalism to support a policy because it prevents other people from harming themselves. The hard question is if a policy may subject *me* to paternalism, if I accept it because of the good it will do others. It seems we can go either way. On the one hand, the policy may count as involving paternalism for me because it interferes with me and I do not find that the interference is made worthwhile by any benefit to me. On the other hand, the policy may count as involving no paternalism, because I do nevertheless welcome it.

It seems likely that on most specifications of the will component, most people would welcome product safety regulation on the level common in the European Union. For them, the regulation will not involve paternalism. However, there are certainly some people who do not welcome regulation, and with whom the regulation is interference, for some or all of the reasons pointed out in the previous section. Product safety regulation, therefore, amounts to unwelcome interference with some people, but not with others.

Good

If a policy amounts to unwelcome interference, it may involve paternalism. For there to be paternalism, however, the interference must be in some sense for

---

[13] This difference has been emphasized in recent calls for a public health ethics distinguished from traditional bioethics, see e.g. Ronald Bayer and Amy L. Fairchild, 'The genesis of public health ethics', *Bioethics*, 18/6 (2004): 473-92.

[14] This is in line with Dworkin's (p. 69) argument that without paternalism, 'individuals [...] may need the use of compulsion to give effect to their collective judgement of their own interest by guaranteeing each individual compliance by the others'.

the good of those interfered with.[15] We tend to think of paternalism as residing in actions, including complex state actions–policies. The good component then functions as a condition on which actions qualify as paternalistic. This is anyway how paternalism is defined in the philosophical literature. Unwelcome interferences are typically said to be paternalistic if they are *motivated* by the good of the person interfered with, or, less commonly, if they are *justified* by the good of this person.[16] However, actions are often motivated, as well as justified, by several different reasons. While this complexity is sometimes acknowledged, the solutions are unsatisfactory. Actions are typically counted as paternalistic when their rationale is solely,[17] or mainly,[18] the good of the person interfered with, or to the extent[19] that this is their rationale. These standard interpretations are ill-suited for distinguishing those morally problematic aspects of paternalism that liberal anti-paternalists are concerned with. The essence of paternalism is the invocation (or acceptance) of the good of a person as a reason for unwelcome interference with her, regardless of the relative strength of this reason as compared to other reasons for the same interference.[20]

When we call a policy paternalistic, this should be interpreted merely as a convenient way to say that it *involves* paternalism, in the sense that the policy is interfering, unwelcome, and that the good of some people who are subject to this unwelcome interference is invoked as a reason for the policy. If we want to distinguish the paternalistic content of a situation more precisely, we must accept that policies are not paternalistic as such, but only in combination with certain reasons. The most obvious and sensible reason for introducing product safety regulation is to protect people from the risk of harm from unsafe products. However, there could be other reasons. A corrupt politician might push for regulations because they favour certain manufacturers. A more altruistic and far-sighted politician may propose regulations because they would stimulate technological innovation, spilling over into other areas. The invocation of these reasons for the policy may be more or less appropriate, but is not paternalistic, regardless of whether or not

15 Seana Shiffrin ['Paternalism, unconscionability doctrine, and accommodation', *Philosophy and Public Affairs*, 29/3 (2000): 215-17] takes an uncommon stand on this issue and argues that acting out of disrespect for a person's judgement or agency is paternalistic regardless of whether or not it is for the good of the person.

16 Or possibly both, as proposed by Peter De Marneffe, 'Avoiding Paternalism', *Philosophy and Public Affairs*, 34/1 (2006): 73-4.

17 E.g. Gerald Dworkin, 'Paternalism', *Stanford Encyclopedia of Philosophy*, ed. Edward N. Zalta (Winter 2002 Edition). Available at: http://plato.stanford.edu/archives/win2002/entries/paternalism/ (accessed July 2007).

18 E.g. Archard, 'Paternalism defined': pp. 38-39.

19 E.g. John Kleinig, *Paternalism* (Manchester: Manchester University Press, 1983): p. 12.

20 For a more detailed argument for this interpretation of paternalism, see Kalle Grill, 'The normative core of paternalism', *Res Publica*, 13/4 (2007): 441-58.

avoidance-of-harm reasons are invoked for the same policy. Similarly, what is paternalistic about involuntary psychiatric treatment is invoking the good of the patient as a reason for treatment, rather than the treatment as such; what is paternalistic about drug criminalization is the invocation of the good of (potential) drug users as a reason for criminalization and punishment, not the criminalization itself; and so on for other policies. We should insist on interpreting paternalism in terms of the invocation of reasons because this, unlike standard action-focused accounts, distinguishes precisely that aspect of policy-making and implementation that is resisted by anti-paternalism.

There is an important complication to be noted in many person cases. Even if a policy interferes with a person and is unwelcome, this may not be enough to make the invocation of her good as a reason for that policy paternalistic. This is because a policy that affects many may promote the good of each by interfering with the others. This is typically the case for policies that we do not think of as involving paternalism, such as laws against theft, assault and murder. These laws restrict the options available to all and may plausibly be unwelcome for some people. There are thus people that are protected by these laws but for whom these laws amount to an unwelcome interference. These people are not, however, protected through the unwelcome interference *with them*, but rather through interference with others, who are not allowed to harm them. Similarly, product safety regulation may to some extent protect people from risks of harm through the interference with other people, as noted above. I may oppose regulation and regulation may be interfering for me, yet when I benefit from the fact that my neighbour is not allowed to buy a dangerous lawnmower that could explode next to my garden table, this benefit occurs as a result of interference with her and not with me. Invoking this benefit to me as a reason for the policy is therefore not paternalism. As we saw in the previous section, restricting the options of others to harm me may in some cases be an interference also with me, as when others are prohibited from selling me dangerous or unhealthy products. The point is that regardless of how we specify interference, we must count as paternalistic only the invocation of a person's good for an action that achieves that good through interference *with her*.

The Moral Status of Paternalism

A great advantage of interpreting paternalism in terms of the invocation of reasons is that we may distinguish different kinds of reasons and consider for each kind whether its invocation is paternalistic or not. Based on such an analysis we may then approach the important normative question of how to evaluate different forms of paternalism. The two main kinds of reasons to consider are arguably psychologically motivating reasons, or motives, and justificatory reasons. Motives cause and explain the actions they are motives for, while justificatory reasons justify, or contribute to the justification of, actions they are reasons for. We could also, however, focus our attention on officially-stated reasons, or reasons invoked in some other context.

Resistance to paternalism may take somewhat different forms depending on what kind of reasons are invoked paternalistically. In terms of justification, anti-paternalism may most obviously be interpreted as a restriction on what reasons should count when we evaluate actions. The liberal anti-paternalist is not necessarily opposed to policies interfering with you. Whether an unwelcome interference is acceptable or right overall may depend on several considerations. What the anti-paternalist claims is that your good is not one of these considerations. We may say that this kind of reason is *invalid* as a reason for this kind of policy. In terms of motives, there may similarly be several reasons why a policy-maker may want to interfere with you against your will. According to anti-paternalism, your good should not be among those reasons. We may say that this motive is *inappropriate* for this kind of policy. As we have seen, having an inappropriate motive does not exclude the possibility of being motivated also by other reasons, which in themselves may be impeccable to the anti-paternalist and which may make the interference in one way commendable.[21]

Given that there are potentially many kinds of reasons, including different interpretations of what counts as a motive and a justification, there is room for a large number of mixed positions on the moral status of paternalism. However, the two end-point strategies are perhaps the most coherent ones. These are general anti-paternalism and the full rejection of anti-paternalism. General anti-paternalism holds that paternalism is never acceptable, neither in motive nor in evaluation, nor in any other kind of reason. In evaluating the desirability of product safety regulation, to determine whether or not it should be introduced, or continued, anti-paternalism directs us to disregard good that will come about through unwelcome interference. The idea of disregarding the interests of some affected people is straightforward, and common in public policy evaluation. We commonly disregard the interests of non-citizens, non-residents and future generations. Similarly, we could disregard the interests in health and safety of those people for which regulation would be an unwelcome interference.

Anti-paternalism is a typically non-consequentialist position. Non-consequentialism holds that, when a moral right or duty is at stake, other considerations are excluded or become irrelevant. Only within the side constraints set by rights and duties may we consider a broader set of more or less worthy

21 There could be moderate anti-paternalist positions that do not completely disregard certain reasons, but rather discount them in some fashion. This seems for example to be the position of Louis Groarke in 'Paternalism and egregious harm', *Public Affairs Quarterly*, 16/3 (2002): 203-30. Discounting a reason can not be equivalent to simply attributing to the reason a low degree of importance in relation to other reasons, since the moral status of paternalism does not tell us anything about the relative importance of different reasons.

aims.[22] Some degree of anti-paternalism therefore forms a natural part of any system of rights or duties where there is no duty to protect or benefit people through unwelcome interference with them, and no right of people to be so protected or benefited. If people have a moral right to buy and sell unsafe products, and there is no conflicting right to be protected against the dangers of such products, that settles the matter against regulation. *No* other considerations than rights and duties are valid, and the avoidance of harm is simply one of these other considerations. This, however, is not a specifically anti-paternalist position. Anti-paternalism can be incorporated into a non-consequentialist theory in full through the right not to be interfered with against one's will for one's good, or in other words the right not to have one's good count as a reason for unwelcome interference. Such a right is general and holds for all unwelcome interference, regardless of whether or not there is a more substantial right to do or have something.

By telling us to disregard certain reasons in making all things considered judgements, anti-paternalism introduces a level of normative consideration that is prior to the common comparison and weighing of reasons. It may be argued that this framework makes moral judgement unnecessarily complicated, or that it unjustifiably attributes to some reasons a special trumping quality.[23] From a broadly consequentialist perspective, there are no reason-regulating principles. Moral rights and duties may be invoked as reasons, but their relative importance must always be measured against the importance of other considerations. To reject anti-paternalism is to hold that all reasons should be admitted into the process of comparing and weighing reasons. No commitment is thereby made concerning the relative importance of different kinds of reasons. The rejection of anti-paternalism is perfectly consistent with strong opposition to policies involving paternalism. Resistance to product safety regulation may take the form of insisting on the value of self-determination or autonomy, and on the greater importance of these considerations relative to the minimizing of risks and promotion of health. The five reasons for holding product safety regulation to be interfering, considered above, can count as reasons against regulation, without trumping or making invalid what reasons there are *for* regulation. If we reject anti-paternalism, liberal values can simply be assigned whatever relative importance we think they deserve, save perhaps infinite importance (which would in effect amount to anti-paternalism).

The rejection of anti-paternalism is furthermore consistent with the use of anti-paternalism-like rules of thumb. Rules of thumb that regulate what reasons to consider may for example arise through the expectations we attach to certain social roles. We should arguably put our private interests aside when we act as representatives for some organization or agency, even if these interests are normally

22 See e.g. Frances Kamm, 'Rights', in Jules Coleman and Scott Shapiro (eds), *The Oxford Handbook of Jurisprudence and Philosophy of Law* (Oxford: Oxford University Press, 2002).

23 Feinberg [*Harm to Self*, p. 26] explicitly calls autonomy a 'moral trump card'.

appropriate motives for action.[24] This moral demand is merely instrumental, however, and does not mean that our private interests lose their normative importance. Rather, the private interests of all are best promoted if we sometimes disregard our own interests. Perhaps, similarly, policy makers should sometimes put aside the interests of people facing unwelcome interference, because this is expedient. It may be that our interests in freedom from interference in some area is so great, and our other interests so small or difficult to ascertain, that the risk of error would be too great to make the effort of considering all affected interests worthwhile, or that it would simply be a waste of resources. Anti-paternalist rules of thumb will only be motivated, however, in areas where it is both wasteful to even consider and estimate all affected interests, and where this is not obvious without a rule of thumb. In view of our great interest in health, and the vast resources available for making and implementing policy in modern welfare states, such areas may be hard to find in the public health context.

Conclusion

Paternalism is the invocation of the good of a person as a reason for unwelcome interference with her. To the extent that product safety regulation amounts to unwelcome interference with some people, invoking the health of these people as a reason for such regulation is paternalism. Anti-paternalism requires that we disregard these reasons. Rejecting anti-paternalism means considering all relevant reasons for and against regulation, without first discarding some as invalid or inappropriate. While anti-paternalism is wide-spread and inherent in the liberal tradition, liberal values need not trump other values in order to be attributed great importance.

Are the *General Product Safety Regulations 2005* a good or justified policy? This would seem to depend on its effects in terms of public health, the restriction and expansion of options, the frustration and satisfaction of preferences, and other relevant values. We should not accept the classification of a public health policy as 'paternalistic' to tell against it, without further argument. The paternalistic content of the situation must be distinguished and the moral status of paternalism must be decided in light of what this content is. Hopefully, this contribution has provided some analytical tools for making such distinctions and decisions.[25]

---

[24] This and other motives for disregarding reasons are discussed by Thomas Scanlon in *What We Owe to Each Other* (Cambridge, MA: Harvard University Press, 1998), 51-2.

[25] This text was completed during a four-month visit to University of California San Diego, financed by the Swedish Foundation for International Cooperation in Research and Higher Education. Thanks to Richard Arneson for our many discussions on paternalism and anti-paternalism during that visit, to Niklas Möller for comments on an early draft, and to the editor of this book for comments on a later draft.

Chapter 10
Newborn Screening and Choosing Whether to Know

Niels Nijsingh
Utrecht University, Netherlands

Sometimes the emergence of new technologies presents us with unexpected problems. An interesting example is the finding of unsought information in newborn screening. The 'accidental' detection of diseases raises the question of what to do with this information. We may wonder whether parents should know about diseases that are detected, particularly when this information is of small practical value. A large number of problems arise when we ask ourselves this question. I will focus here on the question of to what extent parents have a right to choose what information they receive. I will argue that a right to autonomous choice provides no basis for such a right.

Newborn Screening for MCADD and MADD

Newborn screening is performed in a large number of countries all over the world. The participation rate is generally very high; nearly every child in the industrialized world is screened for congenital diseases in the first week after birth. The programmes in different countries started out with a small number of diseases, but gradually most countries have expanded their programmes. Whereas at first screening was mostly performed solely on Phenylketonuria (PKU), new technologies have made it possible to screen for a large variety of diseases. One of the technological developments that caused a minor revolution in the field of newborn screening has been the introduction of tandem mass spectrometry (MS/MS).[1]

MS/MS makes it possible to screen for several dozens of amino, organic and fatty acid disorders, in a relatively cheap and efficient manner. One of the diseases that may be screened for is MCADD (Medium-chain acyl-CoA-dehydrogenase deficiency). MCADD is a metabolic disease that causes lethargy, vomiting and

---

1 See for instance T.H. Zytkvicz, E.F. Fitzgerald, D. Marsden, C.A. Larson, V.E. Shih, D.M. Johnson, A.W. Strauss, A.M. Comeau, R.B. Eaton and G.F. Grady, 'Tandem mass spectrometric analysis for amino, organic and fatty acid disorders in newborn dried blood spots: A two-year summary from the New England newborn screening program', *Clinical Chemistry*, 47/11 (2006): 1945-55.

can possibly result in a coma. Given its prevalence, its treatability and the fact that MCADD can easily be detected, it would be easy to annually save several lives in a medium sized country.[2] Furthermore, the treatment is relatively easy and cheap.[3] Therefore many countries have considered screening for MCADD and some have already implemented screening.

Screening for MCADD by way of MS/MS, however, has a peculiar side-effect: it generates information not only on MCADD, but also on MADD (Multiple-chain acyl-CoA-dehydrogenase deficiency).[4] MADD is a very rare digestive disease, related to MCADD and other amino acid deficiencies. Although patients with milder forms of MADD may respond to riboflavin and L-carnitine, and variable results have been obtained by implementing dietary restrictions, the complexity of the disease make the prognosis for more serious forms very bleak. For this reason it is generally considered to be untreatable, although not necessarily fatal. Knowledge of a positive test result is therefore seen by at least some parents to be a mere burden. Nevertheless, we can imagine that some *would* like to know that their child has a potentially serious condition. Both positions seem to have something to say for them.

Newborn screening for MCADD raises the question what to do with the 'by-product'—the information on MADD. Is it justifiable to simply discard this information, or do we have a duty to preserve any medical information that we stumble upon, even if it is of no practical use? Or should we perhaps abandon MCADD-screening altogether? What are the implications for the informed consent procedure?

Each of these questions is complex in its own right, and I can not elaborate on them all in this paper. Instead, I want to focus on an issue that plays a role in the background of several debates on screening and genetic testing and that comes to the fore in this specific case. This is the question whether people—in this case parents—have a *right to choose* what information they receive. I will argue that there is no such trumping right and that in some situations it is legitimate to withhold or discard information without prior permission. First, to sketch the scene, I will give a quick overview of the issue of informed consent in newborn screening.

---

[2] See S.S. Wang, P.M. Fernhoff, W.H. Hannon and M.J. Khoury, 'Medium chain acyl-CoA dehydrogenase deficiency human genome epidemiology review', *Genetics in Medicine* 1/7 (1999): 332-9.

[3] See for example U. Nennstiel-Ratzel, S. Arenz, E.M. Maier, et al., 'Reduced incidence of severe metabolic crisis or death in children with medium chain acyl-CoA dehydrogenase deficiency homozygous for c.985A>G identified by neonatal screening', *Molecular Genetics and Metabolism* 85 (2005): 157-9.

[4] I use MCADD and MADD as an example here, but there are other examples of screening that generate unsought information. In some respects, a very different example is screening for CF, which can give information on the carrier status of the child.

Informed Consent

Given that there may be reasons for knowing and reasons for not knowing whether your child has MADD, what are the implications for the informed consent procedure? I do not have the space here to go into this question very thoroughly, but before moving on to the main question of this paper, I will just make some brief observations.

The current approach in most countries to newborn screening is to have a rather minimal informed consent procedure. This ensures a high uptake and can be justified by pointing to the clear benefits and little harm for the screened children. However, when expansion of the screening programme provides us with data on diseases for which the benefits are less clear and there may even be harm in knowing, this justification falls away, which raises the question how to offer screening when the results are more controversial. A possible answer is that such an expansion calls for a full or proper informed consent procedure, that is, parents should be aware not only of the possibilities of screening for MCADD but also of the possibility of detecting MADD, and should be allowed to make their own decision on whether they would like to know if their child has MADD. This will not do, however.

It is easy to see that expansion of the newborn screening programme with diseases such as MADD will demand a larger effort by parents to understand the information offered. More and more complex information needs to be submitted to the parents. Given the fact that even currently many parents indicate that they do not know what they agreed to when they agreed to screening,[5] it is not far-fetched to suppose that a proper informed consent procedure is not feasible for an extended programme. Furthermore, such a procedure is likely to be much more costly and time-consuming for all involved. I believe that these considerations give reason to believe that such a programme may be overly burdensome. This problem is all the more pressing, because the diseases we are dealing with are generally very rare. The burdens on an overall healthy population will therefore quickly exceed the acceptable level.[6]

Suppose that this is true and proper informed consent for a newborn screening programme containing MADD is unfeasible and even burdensome. The tempting conclusion to draw is that therefore expansion of newborn screening with MADD

---

[5] See for example, E. Campbell and L.F. Ross, 'Parental attitudes and beliefs regarding the genetic testing of children', *Community Genet,* 8/2 (2005): 94-102. Also: E. Hosli, S. Detmar, N. Dijkstra, N. Nijsingh and M. Verweij, 'Parental preferences towards expanding the neonatal screening programme' (Leiden: TNO Quality of Life, forthcoming).

[6] See N. Nijsingh, 'Informed consent and the expansion of newborn screening', in A. Dawson and M. Verweij (eds), *Ethics, Prevention and Public Health* (Oxford: Oxford University Press, 2007). See also A. Dawson, 'Informed consent: bioethical ideal and empirical reality', in M. Häyry and T. Takala, *Bioethics and Social Reality* (Amsterdam, New York: Rodopi, 2005), on the empirical limits of informed consent.

has itself become problematic. This would imply that, since there is no way of screening for MCADD without also screening for MADD, screening for MCADD becomes problematic too.[7] I would however like to resist this temptation.

A more detailed version of the argument is as follows. From the observation that (1) parents may have reasons to want to know whether their child has MADD as well as reasons not to and (2) the fact that this information is available, it would then be argued that (3) they have a right to choose whether to know whether their child in fact has MADD. (4) This right should be safeguarded by a proper informed consent procedure. However, (5) informed consent is not feasible, nor desirable, particularly for an expanded programme. Therefore, (6) adding MADD to the screening programme infringes upon the right to autonomous choice and (7) a screening programme that provides us with information on MADD is not acceptable.

I want to stress that I am not interested here in questions about the desirability of screening for MADD or MCADD, but instead I want to focus on the third step of this particular argument. I will reject this premise and argue that there no such thing as a (trumping) right to choose which information is conveyed.

The Right to Choice

The previous argument derives the force of its conclusion ('not acceptable') from the trumping character of the right to choice. If the right to choice were just one consideration among many, this conclusion could not be derived, but instead any conclusion ought to be determined in the light of all ethically-relevant aspects. I have no principled problems with this weaker variant of the right to choose information, as I will illustrate below. Those who affirm a right to choose information, however, will generally hold that infringements of this right constitute an infringement of autonomous choice. They will say that people should make their own choices when their health is concerned and that to disclose or withhold information without prior permission is paternalistic, and therefore wrong. This is the strong claim I will be concerned with in this section.

Note that it is not the medical part of the procedure that is the object of choice here. I am assuming that the child will be screened for diseases other than MADD or MCADD anyway, but the question is whether parents should be given a choice to receive the particular information that the screening for MCADD may produce. If

[7] A solution would of course be to screen for MCADD and simply discard information on MADD. This is actually the general procedure in some countries. It is possible to conduct the MS/MS in such a manner that the information need not be actively discarded, but simply 'remains inside the machine'. However, this does not meet standards of informed consent because in this procedure parents remain unaware that this information is available. This matter raises the issue of what the meaning and importance of the notion of 'availability' is. Unfortunately, I do not have the space to get into that interesting topic here.

information is available on the health of a child that is not of therapeutic relevance, does the right to autonomous choice give parents a right to choose whether to receive this information? What sort of right would this be?

There are two opposite ways to infringe upon a right to choose information, either by unsolicited disclosure of information, or by withholding of information without consent. A right to choose information therefore implies both a positive claim-right to know, as well as a negative claim-right not to know. These rights correspond respectively to the duty to inform and the duty not to disclose.

This raises the question 'to know *what*'?[8] A *general* right to know or not to know is not a probable candidate, since in everyday life it constantly occurs that all sorts of information is being disclosed without prior permission, not to mention all the information that is *not* being disclosed to us. It would be implausible to claim that every bit of trivial information I receive or do not receive without prior consent would be an infringement of my right to autonomous choice. So a proponent of a right to choose information should narrow down the scope of the general claim. One way to do this, is to point out that the type of information we are considering when we talk about newborn screening is personal medical information.

A problem that the proponent faces after this narrowing down, is that in the case of newborn screening the one screened and the one who receives the information are not the same person. Since the child is incompetent, and uncomprehending, it is the parents who have the right to choice, and who receive the information. At first sight this observation seems to seriously weaken the argument for a right to choice, but this need not necessarily be so. It is generally acknowledged that there is such a thing as parental autonomy and that this limits government intervention. Parents have a liberty—and even a duty—to make choices for their children, under the condition that these choices do not harm the infant.[9] It is not obvious in the case of choosing for or against being informed on MADD that the child will be harmed. Therefore, the right to choice may still be defended on the ground that this type of decision belongs to the private sphere. This then is the main question of this paper: 'is there a right of the individual parents to decide whether to receive information on the health status of their children, specifically whether their child is affected with MADD?'.

As several authors have shown, there is no moral duty to receive information about the health status of one's child, when this information is of little use.[10] It has

8 See R. Chadwick, 'The philosophy of the right to know and the right not to know', in R. Chadwick, M. Levitt and D. Shickle, *The Right to Know and the Right not to Know* (Aldershot: Ashgate, 1997).

9 A. Dawson, 'The "Best Interests" argument and childhood vaccination', *Bioethics*, 19/2 (2005): 187-205.

10 See for example, T. Takala, 'The right to genetic ignorance confirmed', *Bioethics* 13/3-4 (1999): 288-93; T. Takala, 'Genetic ignorance and reasonable paternalism', *Theoretical Medicine and Bioethics* 22/5 (2001): 485-91; and J. Husted, 'Autonomy and a right not to know', in Chadwick et al., *The Right to Know and the Right not to Know.*

further been argued that since there is no such thing as a duty to attain information on your child's health, and that refusing information can be a reasonable thing to do, there is a claim-right to choose the information that will be conveyed. But this does not follow, at least not directly. It has to be shown that not giving people a choice in this issue is an infringement of autonomous choice. For example Tuija Takala implicitly moves from the one claim to the other. She criticizes a conception of reasonability, which she rightly argues to be too narrow, and from there on switches to the charge of paternalism: 'It seems that by accepting the rhetorics of 'what a reasonable person would do', we re-introduce the practice of paternalism to medical ethics'.[11]

Takala argues that there are mutually exclusive, reasonable conceptions of what information is beneficial to the subject. Therefore, she argues, it would be paternalistic to force people to take note of this information. I agree with her that it may be reasonable to refuse information in relation to ones child's health. I do not agree, however, with the stronger claim Takala defends, which is that therefore parents have a right to *choose* not to know, and that to do otherwise is to infringe upon the right to autonomous choice.

In order to complete this argument, she would have to argue that the choice of the type of information that we are concerned with here should be left to the individual. In other words, she has to show that self-determining individuals have a moral right to make their own choices as to what information they want to receive. I think this step is inherently problematic.

Against a Right to Choose Information

I will here present an argument for the thesis that knowledge cannot be the object of autonomous choice, and that therefore there is no right to choice infringed when there is no proper informed consent.[12] This is, admittedly, a strong claim, which will be modified to some extent in the next section.

When thinking about the notion of choosing to know the result of a newborn screening test, a peculiarity comes to the fore. The choosing whether to know is only an issue when it is presumed that there *is* something to know, in this case that the result of the test is positive. On the other hand, it is not necessary to consider all the negative test results. In other words, when I consider the question 'would I like to know if my child had MADD?', I am not asking a general question on the health status of the child, but instead I am considering the hypothesis that my child has *this* disorder. Parents generally do not mind knowing or not knowing that their child does *not* have a disease. Therefore, the problems of disclosing

[11] See T. Takala, 'Genetic ignorance and reasonable paternalism', p. 490.

[12] I think this argument does not just work when applied to newborn screening, but also for adult screening.

or withholding information do not arise until there is something to disclose or withhold, in this case a positive test result.

There is thus an asymmetry between the situation in which there is a positive test result and that in which the result comes back as negative. This asymmetry is reflected by the fact that every newborn screening programme—at least the ones I know of—does not return the result of the test, unless it is a positive result.

But this means that a crucial part of the information is missing when one deliberates on the question whether one wants to know. When one 'chooses to know' the object of knowledge is principally beyond your grasp. One cannot choose to know or not to know *that* a certain proposition is true, because that would imply that one already knows that this is true. The best thing we can do when we 'choose to know' is hypothetically wonder: '*if* my child had this or that disease, *would* I like to know?'.

This aspect sets the choosing of information apart from other types of choices. When confronted with a choice to undergo surgery we try to inform ourselves as much as we think sufficient and then, given this epistemic state, we make a decision. Of course, there are no guarantees on the outcome of a surgery, and for some decisions there is a large degree of uncertainty, but the difference should be clear: in the case of choosing to know it is precisely the epistemic state that is at stake. There is therefore no way, not even theoretically, to be sufficiently informed on the choice you are making.

When I decide to find out the truth of a trivial piece of information, this is generally not a problem. Either I look it up, or I do not, and on the whole no one will be worse off either way. However, when the information is considered potentially harmful, the situation becomes different. The diagnosis of MADD is harmful just because it is a positive test result. Since there is an asymmetry between a positive and a negative result, nobody would claim that a right to choice is infringed when it is disclosed that a child *does not* have MADD.

Once this is acknowledged, it is a small step to show that not giving someone a choice to know cannot be an infringement of autonomous choice, because the very same information that is the object of choice would be the relevant fact in deciding whether to know. And then there is no ground from where we can determine what we would and what we wouldn't like to know. Since the result of the MADD screening test is already 'known' to the screening authorities this situation must be interpreted as one where the authorities hold information that may be decisive in determining what choice to make. How could this be a situation where the subject is said to make an autonomous decision?

This argument presupposes a distinction between the object of choice, and that which enables a choice. The very notion of autonomous choice already implies being informed. Therefore, the argument continues, when the information that is needed for making a choice is the same as that which is the object of choice, there can be no right to choose this information. This may seem like playing with words, or nitpicking, but I think in fact that the argument points out that there is something strange about the phrase 'choosing to know'. I believe that generally when we use this phrase in the context of screening, we use it as roughly synonymous for 'choosing to have a (specific) test done'. But in the case of screening for MCADD/ MADD, the question is not whether the test should be done, but what information parents want to get out of it. And on this question, I would hold, it is implausible to say that people can be self-determining.

I believe that this argument establishes that there is no trumping right to choose to be informed on a specific piece of information. If information cannot be said to be the object of autonomous choice, we can clearly not demand of a screening programme that the autonomous choice of the individual is respected. It follows that from a moral perspective, a proper informed consent procedure is not necessarily required for this type of choice. This point can however easily lead to misunderstandings. Therefore I try to take away some of the possible misunderstandings below.

Where Does This Argument Lead Us?

The notion of a choice of information depends on the idea of being able to 'control the outward flow of information',[13] thus managing data that are principally out of grasp. This idea is a phantasm. Subjects are relatively helpless in determining what they would and what they wouldn't like to know. The 'flow of information' is a complex, intricate weave of very different types of strands. The different types of information vary in relevance, certainty, practical use, and so on. Controlling this flow implies also controlling the flows of everything we do not know. This does not mean that anything goes in the field of information policy. It does follow however that the proponent of the right not to know has a much weaker case than it might initially seem. Since there is no case for the position that the absence of a proper informed consent procedure to guarantee the right to choose information necessarily constitutes an infringement of autonomous choice, we will have to look at the desirability of such a procedure on a case by case basis.

Returning to the case of newborn screening, what does this mean for the case of MCADD/ MADD screening? I already noted that we cannot expect of every single parent to make a decision on the testing of their child for hundreds of diseases, most of which are so rare that the most basic information, such as the natural development of the disease, is unknown even to medical science. Naturally, it is possible for parents to reasonably consent or dissent to their child being tested, or being tested for a particular subset of diseases, but it would be wrong to construe this as choosing information.

However, this does not mean that subjects should simply submit to whatever screening authorities think is best for them. Neither would I claim that parents who

---

13 The quote is derived from R. Brownsword, 'An interest in human dignity as the basis for genomic torts', *Washburn Law Journal*, 42/3 (2003): 417. I am not implying that the position I criticize is one he would underwrite, in fact I think he would not.

are informed contrary to their wishes therefore have no reason to complain. Being informed can be very burdensome, and to go against people's preferences for not knowing can—but need not—be morally problematic. And of course, this goes the other way round too. If someone would like to know something and it is withheld, this can be morally problematic.

For this reason there is an argument to be careful in screening for extremely rare and untreatable conditions, such as MADD. The fact that there is no such thing as autonomously choosing to know, in no way implies that all information is or would be welcome, or even that every person would value information in the same way. There is no reason to assume that information, by virtue of being information, will enhance a subject's autonomy or serve its interests.[14] This observation might lead us to the conclusion that it is better to discard information on MADD that surfaces when screening on MCADD. If however the policy is chosen to communicate such findings, we should accept that this will not meet the regular criteria of informed consent.

An element in this argument is the fact that newborn screening concerns a large number of rare diseases. Since there is no reason to suspect that an individual child will be affected with a particular disease, the number of options is very large. The difference with testing for diseases which run in the family, where there is to my opinion no question that the patient's wishes should be respected, should be obvious. To take a well-known example, if someone does not want to be tested for Huntington's disease, that should be the end of the discussion. It would be a mistake, however, to think that this provides a counter-example to the argument in the previous section. Persons who are at risk of being affected with Huntington's are already aware that they are at risk, and therefore 'informed'. While it is impossible to hold that these persons are fully informed, they are significantly *better* informed than persons who consent to newborn screening. Not only in the sense that they are better aware what the disease entails, but also in the sense that they are *in fact* at risk.

Furthermore, there is a case to be made that if a person is tested for Huntington's, a negative finding is not as trivial as in the case of newborn screening. To disclose a negative result for a disease that 'runs in the family' can be burdensome too. We can for example imagine that this causes feelings of guilt towards their next of kin. The idea here is not that the choice whether or not to test for Huntington's is in all ways an autonomous one, but rather that people who have family members that have Huntington's are already trying to find ways to deal with the fact that they and their relatives are at a higher risk of being affected and can therefore not be considered a 'mere negative'. Therefore, there is here a much stronger case

[14] Here I fully agree with, for example, Takala, 'Genetic ignorance and reasonable paternalism' and Husted, 'Autonomy and a right not to know'.

than in the case of newborn screening for being sensitive to and inquiring after the particular individual's wishes.[15]

Information on one's health status tends to be gradual. Informing persons that they are at risk, or a carrier, or affected, or that the first symptoms of a disease are beginning to develop, are all very different types of conveying knowledge. Thus to inform a person can mean very different things in different contexts. However, 'a right to choose information' wrongly suggests that there is a single piece of information 'out there', and that we can either choose to pick it up, or choose not to. In opposition to this I would stress that whether or not informed consent is appropriate depends on other features of the case at hand than merely the question whether a person gets to choose.

By dropping the demand for autonomous choice in newborn screening, I have not claimed that an informed consent procedure for newborn screening is unnecessary or a mere burden. Informed consent procedures have other purposes than just the protection of autonomy. Other considerations are taken in account when assessing the desirability of a particular screening programme, such as privacy and well-being. I do believe that the argument for a right to choice loses its initial force, and that it does not give us a trumping argument against screening for MCADD. Even if a screening programme implies that people do not always get to decide about all the information that is available on the health status of their children, this need not be a decisive argument against this screening. Since we cannot expect parents to control that which is out of reach, it is not necessarily paternalistic not to offer them a choice.[16]

---

15 A complication is of course that since Huntington's disease is an inherited disease, results can affect others too, in a much more direct way than in the case of newborn screening. This should not take away the attention from the point I wish to make, which is that when a disease runs in the family there is already much information available to its members, even before they themselves are tested.

16 I greatly benefited from the comments of Anne van Bergen, Deryck Beyleveld, Bernice Bovenkerk, Angus Dawson, Marie Gaille, Annemarie Kalis, Lonneke Poort and Paul Sollie on earlier drafts of this paper.

Chapter 11
Choosing to Sleep

Benjamin Hale
Colorado University, USA

Lauren Hale
State University of New York, Stony Brook, USA

In a recent article in the *Journal of Public Health* ('Who has time to sleep?') one co-author demonstrated that 'high-risk sleep durations (short-sleeping and long-sleeping) are positively associated with sociodemographic categories associated with poorer health'.[1] Hale's paper has generally been read with the understanding that 'poorer health' is an undesirable objective and that the conclusions of such research are obvious: public policies that encourage populations to practice effective sleep hygiene ought to be encouraged. (The National Sleep Foundation, for instance, offers a set of sleep hygiene tips that derive directly from the observation that better sleep habits are correlated with better health).[2] But this is not necessarily the only implication of such research. It could instead be argued that sleep patterns reveal a necessary connection with other important normative variables, like opportunities to freely will and fulfill life projects.

In this paper we will claim that individual subjects do not have so much control over sleep that it can aptly be characterized as a personal choice; and that normative implications related to public health and sleep hygiene do not necessarily follow from current findings. It should be true of any empirical study that normative implications do not necessarily follow, but we think that many public health sleep recommendations falsely infer these implications from a flawed explanatory account of the decision to sleep: the consumer choice view. This view, which we criticize here, proposes that sleep duration and sleep quality can be understood as one choice among many.

Our strategy will be the following. First we will give a brief overview of the treatment of sleep by empirical researchers, and turn specifically to a linear model of sleep that has been dominant in the past. In this case, Hale (2005)

---

1 L. Hale, 'Who has time to sleep?', *Journal of Public Health*, 27/2 (2005): 205-11.

2 See http://www.sleepfoundation.org/ Sleep hygiene is a term used to refer to a set of sleep-promoting habits such as establishing a regular bedtime routine and schedule, using relaxation techniques before bedtime, limiting sleep to the bedroom, avoiding stimulants and/or large meals before bedtime, exercising regularly but not within one hour of bedtime, limiting light in the bedroom, and keeping the bedroom at a comfortable temperature.

presents innovative methodologies that fly in the face of earlier linear models of the relationship between sleep and sociodemographic variables. We understand models of sleep to be primarily descriptive and to fall into at least two categories: the linear and the curvilinear.[3] Our concerns in this paper, however, relate to explanatory accounts, or views, of what is happening in such models. We will therefore discuss what we will call the 'choice view' (or 'consumer choice view') of sleep, which proposes that one can choose to sleep; versus the 'autonomy view' of sleep, which proposes that sleep tracks autonomy. It will be our position that while the descriptive linear model of sleep does lend itself to the explanatory choice view, the descriptive curvilinear model of sleep challenges the choice view. Instead, the results of the curvilinear model can better be explained by the autonomy view.

It is our primary purpose to argue that although the choice view may be the simplest way to conceive of sleep, it is neither the view that best explains the data, nor the view that best suits a robust picture of the decision to sleep. Following Norman Malcolm, our presupposition will be that sleep cannot adequately be understood as a 'choice' because the subject retires, so to speak, upon falling asleep.[4] It is far more helpful, therefore, to conceive of decisions to sleep as composed of a set of action parameters that the subject sets for himself by deference to practical reasons. In the much bigger picture, though unfortunately not in this short paper, what we argue is that the parameters of sleep-time should be construed as more-or-less flexible options over which one can exercise autonomous control. These parameters constitute the extent of the choice to sleep, and these parameters are frequently shaped by external considerations tied to fulfilment of life projects.

Empirical Research

Literature on Sleep Duration and Health

The simplistic perspective that 'more sleep is always healthier' is called into question by a large body of empirical evidence showing that both ends of the sleep duration distribution are associated with higher morbidity and mortality risks.[5]

[3] As you will see later, we use the term 'curvilinear' to refer to an upside down U-curve in which the optimal amount of sleep ranges between 6.5 and 8.5 hours with the peak being somewhere in between and with those sleep durations outside the optimal being sub-optimal and so tapering near the ends of the distribution. In work by Hale (2005), she does not model a smoothed curve, but rather a 3-category model of duration of sleep for modelling simplicity.

[4] N. Malcolm, 'Dreaming and skepticism', *The Philosophical Review*, 65/1 (1956): 14-37.

[5] A. Tamakoshi and Y. Ohno, 'Self-reported sleep duration as a predictor of all-cause mortality: results from the JACC study, Japan', *Sleep*, 27/1 (2004): 51-4; D.L. Wingard

Studies repeatedly show that 6.5-7.5 hours of sleep on an average weeknight is associated with the lowest risk of all-cause mortality.[6] In one large study, controlling for demographic characteristics, health behaviours, prior health conditions and medication use, it was shown that sleeping either a long or short amount increases the relative risk of all-cause mortality by up to 40 per cent.[7] Interpretation of the findings of greater mortality with long-sleep durations is controversial. The studies are often based on self-reported sleep time, and some people, perhaps those with unrecognized health conditions, report sleep duration based on the hours they spend in bed, rather than actual sleep time. Long-sleep duration may also be a marker for sleep apnea, a sleep disorder that is associated with breathing pauses that profoundly fragment sleep. However, since the relationship between long-sleep and poor health is so commonly observed, we suggest that there may be something more fundamental, such as socioeconomic factors or individual autonomy, underlying the relationship that is more important than measurement error or confounding comorbidities.

Relationship between Sleep Duration and Socioeconomic Factors

To support our argument, we are interested in how socioeconomic factors are correlated with short, mid-range, and long-sleep durations. In 2005, Hale introduced a model in which sleep is conceived of as having two suboptimal categories (short and long-sleep duration) and one optimal sleep duration (mid-range sleep duration).[8] This is in contrast to previous models of sleep in which

---

and L.F. Berkman, 'Mortality risk associated with sleeping patterns among adults', *Sleep*, 6/2 (1983): 102-7; A.I. Qureshi, W.H. Giles, J.B. Croft and D.L. Bliwise, 'Habitual sleep patterns and risk for stroke and coronary heart disease: a 10-year follow-up from NHANES I', *Neurology*, 48/4 (1997): 904-11; S.R. Patel, N.T. Ayas, M.R. Malhotra, et al., 'A prospective study of sleep duration and mortality risk in women', *Sleep*, 27/3 (2004): 440-44; D.F. Kripke, L. Garfinkel, D.L. Wingard, et al., 'Mortality associated with sleep duration and insomnia', *Archives of General Psychiatry*', 59/2 (2002): 131-6; N.T. Ayas, D.P. White, W.K. Al-Delaimy, et al., 'A prospective study of self-reported sleep duration and incident diabetes in women', *Diabetes Care*, 26/2 (2003): 380-84, N.T. Ayas, D.P. White, J.E. Manson, et al., 'A prospective study of sleep duration and coronary heart disease in women', *Archives of Internal Medicine*, 163/2 (2003): 205-9; D.F. Kripke, R.N. Simons, L. Garfinkel and E.C. Hammond, 'Short and long-sleep and sleeping pills. Is increased mortality associated?', *Archives of General Psychiatry*, 36/1 (1979): 103-16.

6 Tamakoshi and Ohno, 'Self-reported sleep duration as a predictor of all-cause mortality: results from the JACC study, Japan'; Wingard and Berkman, 'Mortality risk associated with sleeping patterns among adults'; Kripke, et al., 'Mortality associated with sleep duration and insomnia'.

7 Kripke, et al., 'Mortality associated with sleep duration and insomnia'.

8 Hale, 'Who has time to sleep?'.

sleep is allowed to be a continuous variable.[9] This difference in classification is an improvement in that it not only better fits with the empirical relationship between sleep and health described above, but also because it better suits a plausible view of the nature of the decision to sleep.

Description studies using a curvilinear model of sleep duration There are only a few studies that have explicitly investigated social factors and their relationship to short, mid-range, and long-sleepers.[10] Hale[11] uses time-use data from four cross-sectional datasets[12] and estimates a multinomial logistic regression equation on the amount of sleep reported for the 24-hour period of the time-use diary. The three outcome categories are short-sleep (<6.5 hours), mid-range sleep (6.5-8.5 hours), and long-sleep (>8.5 hours). Hale controls for factors such as calendar year, marital status, gender, educational status, employment, minutes of television watched, age and age-squared. In a similar set of analyses, Hale and Do[13] use survey data from the *National Health Interview Study* (NHIS). In these models, they include additional variables to the ones above including race and neighbourhood characteristics. In the third analysis, Adams[14] used data from almost 1,500 respondents in the *Office of National Statistics Omnibus Survey* collected in 1999 in the United Kingdom. Rather than modelling the three categories of sleep duration separately, as done by Hale, Adams used a logistic regression in which the outcome category was a dichotomous variable representing either 6.5-8.5 hours of sleep or not (<6.5 or >8.5).

---

[9] C.D. Jefferson, C.L. Drake, T. Roehrs and T. Roth, 'Sleep habits in healthy normals', *Poster Presentation at the Annual Meetings of the Associated Professional Sleep Society* (2005); D.S. Lauderdale, K.L. Knutson, L.L. Yan, et al., 'Objectively measured sleep characteristics among early-middle-aged adults: the CARDIA study', *American Journal of Epidemiology*, 164/1 (2006): 5-16; P.J. Moore, N.E. Adler, D.R. Williams and J.S. Jackson, 'Socioeconomic status and health: the role of sleep', *Psychosomatic Medicine*, 64/2 (2002): 337-44; J.E. Biddle and D.S. Hamermesh, 'Sleep and the allocation of time', *The Journal of Political Economy*, 98/5 (1990): 922-43.

[10] Hale, 'Who has time to sleep?'; L. Hale and D.P. Do, 'Sleep and the city: an analysis of sleep duration, race, and neighborhood context in the NHIS', *Presented at the Annual Meetings of the Population Association of America* (April 1 2006); J. Adams, 'Socioeconomic position and sleep quantity in UK adults', *Journal of Epidemiology & Community Health*, 60/3 (2006): 267-9.

[11] Hale, 'Who has time to sleep?'.

[12] J. Robinson, S. Bianchi and S. Presser, 'Family interaction, social capital, and trends in time use (FISCT) 1998-1999' (2001); J. Robinson and G. Godbey, *Time for Life: The Surprising Ways Americans Use Their Time* (University Park: Pennsylvania State University, 1999).

[13] Hale and Do, 'Sleep and the city: an analysis of sleep duration, race, and neighborhood context in the NHIS'.

[14] Adams, 'Socioeconomic position and sleep quantity in UK adults'.

Results of curvilinear model of sleep duration Less education is associated with both short and long-sleep duration.[15] One study finds that people without a high school degree are both more likely to be short-sleepers (OR=1.43, $p<0.01$) and long-sleepers (OR=1.61, $p<0.001$) on the weekdays, relative to people with a college degree.[16] The NHIS data show that individuals with a college degree are 21 per cent ($p<0.001$) less likely to be short-sleepers, and 46 per cent ($p<0.001$) less likely to be long-sleepers than those with a high school degree.[17] The Adams study found this to be true of women, but not statistically significant for men.[18]

Unemployment and retirement are both associated with increased risks of long-sleeping. Both Hale studies found that people who are unemployed and retired have an increased likelihood of long-sleeping on the weekdays compared to people who work <36 hours in the week (OR=1.43, $p<0.05$ and OR=1.90, $p<0.01$[19] and OR=1.91, $p<.001$ and OR=1.31,[20] $p<.05$, for unemployment and retirement, respectively).

Marital status is also correlated with sleep duration in a non-linear manner. On the weekdays, relative to being married, separated/divorced (OR=1.29, $p<.05$), widowed (OR=2.04, $p<.001$), and single people (OR=1.61, $p<.001$) are more likely to be short-sleepers compared to married people.[21] Hale and Do[22] find similar relationships in the NHIS in which widowed and divorced people are more likely to be short-sleepers compared to married people controlling for other social characteristics. They also find that single people are more likely to be long-sleepers.[23]

Hale and Do found that controlling for individual characteristics such as education, obesity, smoking behaviours, short- and long-sleep durations are more common in black Americans than in white Americans (OR=1.54, $p<.001$ and OR=1.57, $p<.001$ for short and long-sleeping respectively). A portion of the increased risk of short-sleep duration for blacks can be explained by adding in controls for neighbourhood characteristics (i.e. living in the inner city), but this does not explain all of the effect.

---

15 Hale, 'Who has time to sleep?'; Hale and Do, 'Sleep and the City: An Analysis of Sleep Duration, Race, and Neighborhood Context in the NHIS'; J. Adams,'Socioeconomic position and sleep quantity in UK adults'.

16 Hale, 'Who has time to sleep?'.

17 Hale and Do, 'Sleep and the city: an analysis of sleep duration, race, and neighborhood context in the NHIS'.

18 Adams, 'Socioeconomic position and sleep quantity in UK adults'.

19 Hale, 'Who has time to sleep?'.

20 Hale and Do, 'Sleep and the city: an analysis of sleep duration, race, and neighborhood context in the NHIS'.

21 Hale, 'Who has time to sleep?'.

22 Hale and Do, 'Sleep and the city: an analysis of sleep duration, race, and neighborhood context in the NHIS'.

23 Ibid.

Non-linear relationships are also found between sleep duration and being overweight and smoking patterns. Overweight people are 26 per cent ($p<0.001$) more likely to be short-sleepers and 14 per cent ($p<0.05$) more likely to be long-sleepers than their normal weight counterparts.[24] In addition, current smokers have a 25 per cent increased risk of being a short-sleeper and a 22 per cent increased risk of being a long-sleeper relative to their non-smoking peers.[25]

From the Descriptive to the Explanatory

For the purposes of this paper, then, there are two sets of models at play. One set of models is descriptive and relates to the empirical findings detailed above. These descriptive models describe the relationship between sleep duration and health. The other set of models, or views, is explanatory, in that it seeks to describe the nature of the relationship between the subject's reasoning and sleep. These views seek to characterize the nature of the option to sleep. In our case, we will examine the choice view, which proposes that one can *choose* to sleep, and introduce the autonomy view, which proposes that sleep tracks autonomy. We argue below that the curvilinear model, which we understand to better describe the data, fits more comfortably with the autonomy view than with the choice view. Unfortunately, as with many studies of this nature, both the choice view and the autonomy view can explain the findings in either descriptive model. The difficulty, we will argue, is that the kind of choosing that underwrites the choice view is either inconsistent or incoherent.

Look at the linear model first. On the linear model (Figure 11.1) sleep is understood across a 24-hour horizon, and it is thought that the only negative effects of sleep can result from a lack of sleep. On this view, the optimal amount of sleep is the amount that a body would naturally get, provided that a subject does not interfere with the sleep through some set of decisions (alarm clocks, late nights, and so on).

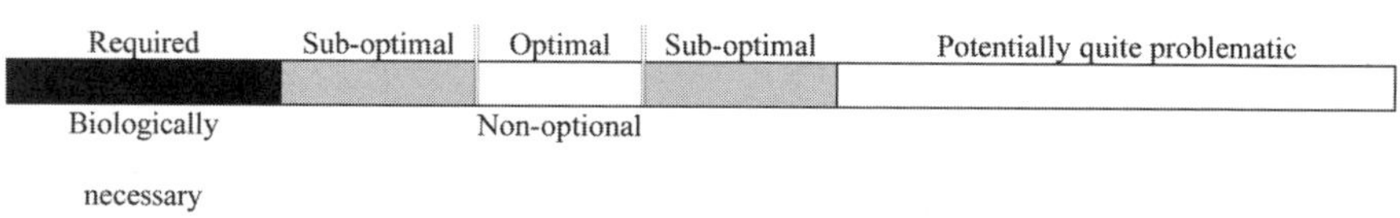

Figure 11.1 The Linear Model

As we explained above, there is another descriptive model that reveals different relationships between subjects, health outcomes, and sleep. This model, pioneered

[24] Ibid.

[25] Ibid.

by Hale, we are calling the curvilinear model (Figure 11.2), because it stipulates that human adults need a certain range of sleep; and that sleep that either falls short of or extends beyond this range of sleep is sub-optimal. In the past, this has been understood as primarily a methodological innovation, but we assert here that it is a methodological innovation with significant descriptive and explanatory force. That is, it not only better describes the relationship of sleep to health factors, but also points to a particular view of how the subject is related to his decision with regard to sleep.

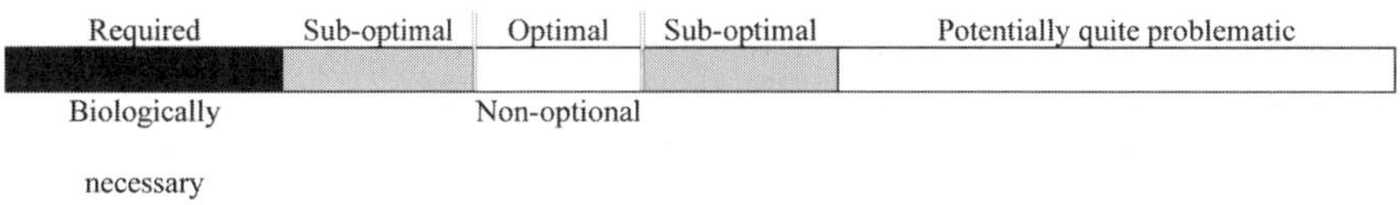

Figure 11.2 The Curvilinear Model

The Choice View

Jeff Biddle and Daniel Hamermesh, both economists, find that the amount of time that one sleeps is 'inversely related to both the wage and time spent in the labour market'.[26] They rightly point out that on most prior models, sleep time was understood primarily as a biological given—a set aside. What they find, however, is that many of our other daily decisions can cut into our sleep time, such that we can effectively choose our sleep schedules.[27] They draw from their research the conclusion that 'sleep is subject to consumer choice and is affected by the same economic variables that affect choices about other uses of time'.[28]

What Biddle and Hamermesh suggest is that one chooses sleep duration based on the value of other possible time-consuming activities. So, one might fill one's days with only a few hours of work, for instance, but this work might be particularly rewarding. Or one might fill one's evenings with family time, and this too might be more rewarding than the sleep that one gets. On Biddle and Hamermesh's consumer choice view of sleep, decisions to sleep are made in such a way that work and other life choices effectively *crowd out* sleep. This view—the choice view (See Figure 11.3)—proposes that the subject's other valued interests

[26] Biddle and Hamermesh, 'Sleep and the allocation of time'.

[27] 'People spend close to one-third of their time sleeping, but it is wrong to view these unconscious hours as a predetermined deduction from their scarce allotment of time. We have shown that at least part of sleep time is a reserve on which people can draw when economic circumstances make other uses of time more attractive. Our results suggest that it is not unusual for people's average daily sleep time to differ by as much as one hour at different times in their adult lives' (Biddle and Hamermesh: 1990).

[28] Ibid.

impinge on the sleep-time of the subject, such that, if the subject so chooses, he can take precious time away from his sleep to engage in other activities.

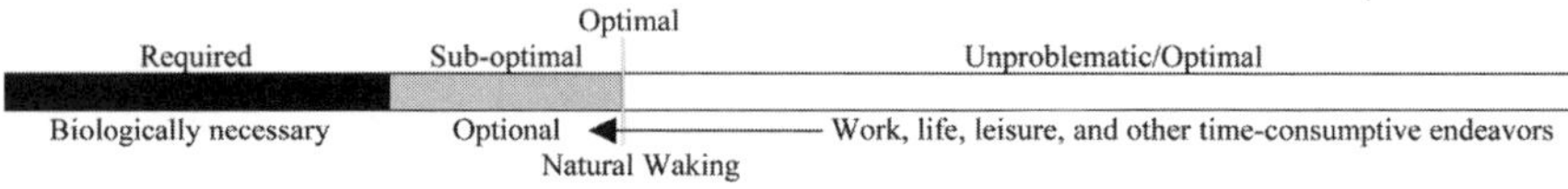

Figure 11.3 The Choice View

Criticism of the Choice View

There is a trivial sense in which one does not choose the amount of time that one sleeps. Ask an insomniac if he has the choice to sleep and you will elicit guffaws. Trivially, then, saying that one has a choice to sleep is like saying that one can will oneself to sleep. This alone might be enough to condemn the choice view, since the empirical data measure the amount of time sleeping and not the amount of time spent trying to get to sleep. But we might also read the position more charitably, and propose that the choice view suggests not that subjects choose the amount of time that they sleep, but only the entry and exit points of their sleep, when they go to bed and when they wake up.

The choice view could withstand the criticism that one cannot will oneself to sleep if framed in this way. Advocates of the view might say, for instance, that psychologically or biologically we have little control over our systems, which is similar to many other choices that we make. Just as we can choose to eat a box of doughnuts but not whether we will get indigestion; just as we can choose to try and get pregnant, but not whether we will, in fact, get pregnant; so too can we choose to try and sleep, but not whether we will, in fact, get to sleep. What we choose, on this view, is to go to bed or to wake at a set hour, not how many hours we sleep. So long as we are not burdened with a pathology like insomnia or sleep apnea—which is a pathology affecting the inside span of our entry and exit points—it makes sense to speak of sleep as a choice. Just as Biddle and Hamermesh suggest, we can shave off hours from our normal sleep schedule to make room for other activities by setting the bedposts of our sleep.

One thing that should be clear, however, is that the choice view depends upon the notion that the subject maintains control of both these entry and exit points. Bodies that sleep for *longer* periods of time than a subject desires—longer periods of time than the body needs—would, on this view, depend upon a body's proclivity to wake on its own, and not on any choice that a subject might make. If a subject plans to head to bed at 12:00, thinking that he will wake naturally by 8:00, but then wakes only at 10:00, such a sleep cycle is unchosen. He has overslept, which he did not choose. In this case, he has long slept.

What the curvilinear model stipulates is that there is such a thing as long-sleeping. If there is such a thing as long-sleeping, then there must be something against which the sleeping is deemed to be long. (Sleeping is deemed to be long when the body sleeps longer than the body needs. Here, long-sleeping is presumed to be unnatural.) And, if there is something against which the sleeping is deemed to be long, then it would appear that it is not the case that some portion of the population chooses what time to wake up.[29] If these people end up sleeping long, then they only *end up* sleeping long, and do not *choose* to sleep long. People can only, reasonably, choose to sleep short, which they can do by placing their will ahead of themselves at the beginning of the night: by asking their partners to jostle them as they snooze or by setting the alarm. As the curvilinear model demonstrates, there are some cases in which people long sleep. Long-sleeping can be a choice no more than the choice to add five inches to a rope of a given length might be a choice.

We might try to remedy the definition of the choice view by employing the suggestion that what we mean by 'choosing' one's entry and exit points is only that one 'allows oneself' to long-sleep. We sometimes speak of our choices this way. But if we do this, then this use of 'choosing' should apply in all instances captured by the choice view, and we can see that this is plainly false. For if this were our meaning when using the description 'choose', choosing to short-sleep would make little sense. We would then also speak of short-sleeping as a sleep duration that we 'just allow'. And this too seems impossible. When we speak of short-sleeping, if we are to speak of choosing short-sleeping and not of pathological short-sleeping (like insomnia), we suggest clearly that we have set premature entry and exit points. What it would mean to allow ourselves to short-sleep would be *to not set up* entry and exit points, but rather just to let sleeping happen as it may. So, either we are not talking about the same kind of 'choice' in the case of both long-sleeping and short-sleeping, and the choice view is inconsistent; or we *are* talking about the same kind of 'choice', which cannot be a choice at all for long-sleepers, and the choice view is incoherent.

And so, the choice view, if it is to withstand the findings of the curvilinear model and the existence of 'long-sleeping', is flawed. There is therefore also a non-trivial sense in which one does not choose to sleep.

The Autonomy View

We are then stuck in a position where we must find another explanation for the decision-making view best associated with sleeping. A reasonably clear position is available to us in the broad body of literature generally associated with talk of autonomy, or self-governance. This body of literature is too broad to justly

---

[29] Remember, the choice view seeks to explain the decision-making behind the data; and so in this sense is also descriptive. It does not propose that one cannot, given knowledge that one's health might be deleteriously affected by long-sleeping, choose to sleep in shorter increments. Rather, it proposes that sleep duration can be understood as a choice; which, in the case of long-sleeping, it cannot. One is effectively always oversleeping.

summarize in a short paper of this nature, but the central idea is that the truly autonomous agent maintains the possibility of freely willing and setting for himself life projects, policies, and practices; and is not coerced or pressured into positions by external forces. One of the most widely accepted ways in which one might be said to acquire this sort of autonomy is by gaining an education. This is the kind of autonomy to which we are referring: autonomy as self-determination.

On our autonomy view, unlike the choice view, it is not the case that the subject selects the entry and exit points of sleep time like one might choose between wine or beer, but rather chooses the *parameters* of sleep time according to a set of life projects in which she is engaged or plans to engage. The autonomy view, we propose, both better explains the data and serves to better characterize the kind of reasoning that goes into decisions about sleep time. Less education, unemployment, and marital status, for instance, are all positively associated with longer and less healthy sleep durations.

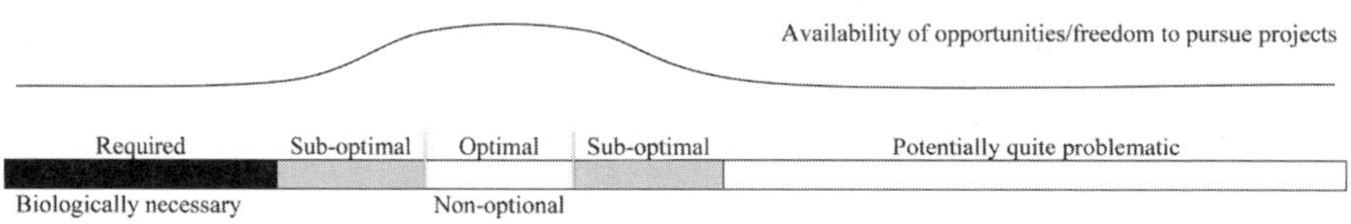

Figure 11.4 The Autonomy View

Due to space limitations, we cannot present the full conceptual argument for the autonomy view here, but do so in a longer version of this paper.[30] Instead we will have to rely on the empirical data presented above to support this claim. In effect, however, we argue elsewhere that reasoning about sleep always maintains a purposive structure, such that decisions about sleep are not appropriately understood as tradeoffs, but rather as purposeful actions taken in order to fulfil projects.[31] In other words, the discrepancy between the views can be explained, in part, by the kind of reasoning that goes into decisions about sleep. On the choice view, decisions about sleep are made via valuations of hours that could either be spent sleeping or doing something else. If I set my entry time at 12:00 and my exit time at 8:00, I am making value decisions based on tasks that I need to accomplish at given times during the day.

30 B. Hale and L. Hale, 'Strange bedfellows: autonomy, ethics, and the sleep of reason', *The annual conference of the Society for Applied Philosophy: The Philosophy of Public Health* (Manchester University, 2006).

31 Hale and Hale, 'Strange bedfellows: Autonomy, ethics, and the sleep of reason'; B. Hale and L. Hale, 'The Decision to Sleep' (forthcoming).

> I'll be at work until 7:00; at the gym from 7:00 until 8:00; out to dinner from 8:00 until 9:00; and at the bar from 9:00 until 12:00. At that point, I'll set my entry point of sleep for 12:00, because that is when I can schedule sleep.

On the autonomy view, the reasoning works according to projects. I do not schedule my sleep according to entry and exit points, but according to what I need of sleep as a whole. In this sense, I say:

> I need roughly seven hours of sleep; and given what I know about my sleep habits; and given what I know about what I need to function at a minimally productive level, if I go to bed at 12:00, I should set my alarm for no earlier than 7:00 in the morning. Or, if I know that I must wake at 6:00, but need at least seven hours of sleep, I must set my bedtime for approximately 11:00.

From the standpoint of what one *does*, this may not appear much different than setting the entry and exit points of sleep. But from a practical reasoning standpoint, this kind of logic has an important practical role to play.

Implications of the Position

The explanatory view that underwrites sleep models has significant implications for the normative conclusions that emerge from these models. For if it is true that sleep tracks autonomy, then it is probably not true that one ought to encourage citizens to value sleep more than they do. Instead, what is probably true is that one ought to encourage *practices* and *projects* that will then promote optimal sleep. In this case it would appear that—because one cannot *choose* to sleep optimally, but instead only sleep optimally when life does not throw obstacles in the way; or sleep optimally only when sleep is for the purpose of some other end; or when opportunities are available to subjects—the correct interpretation of the data is to suggest that, if one desires to improve health by encouraging sleep, one can only do so by ensuring that opportunities for freely willing life projects are distributed as widely as possible.

Moreover, this conclusion suggests that the domain of the public health practitioner is considerably broader than it might at first appear. It is not, in other words, that the public health practitioner can be concerned just with healthy sleep habits, but instead must be concerned with the whole life package. If Hale's curvilinear model suggests that sleep tracks autonomy; and if the objective of the public health official is to promote the health of the public; and if the public is not as healthy as it could be because it is not sleeping optimally; then the following normative conclusion might naturally follow: citizens burdened by other concerns quite independent of their sleeping, but that nevertheless impinge on their sleeping, ought to be *relieved of these concerns*. One must provide opportunities for citizens to better their lives. We cannot argue for this here, but that is a potential implication of this argument.

Conclusion

Our strategy has been first to show that a curvilinear model that recognizes both short and long-sleeping is better suited to the public health data than a linear model. We employed this observation to argue that the choice view is incoherent, which we suggested is revealed by the very idea that there is such a thing as long-sleeping. While it may clearly be the case that one could choose something like short-sleeping, it seems impossible, ignoring the possibility of barbiturate or sleeping pill consumption, to *choose* to long-sleep. Therefore, we suggested, the choice view is flawed; at least so far as explaining the data is concerned. Moreover, we suggested that the choice view attempts to characterize sleep as a choice, where this is clearly both trivially and nontrivially false. One cannot choose to sleep any more than one can will oneself to sleep; and one cannot choose the parameters of sleep time without being either inconsistent or incoherent.

We then suggested that the only coherent position is one that does not conceive of sleep as a choice, but that conceives of the entry and exit points of sleep as a choice, where these are parameters that we can set without the guarantee that our bodies will cooperate. So, we set our alarms, say; and we go to bed at a certain time. That is the kind of choosing that we can do. But what's unique about this kind of choosing is that it does not come with the one-off value characterization: choosing to sleep is not a consumer choice like choosing between wine or beer. Sleep is almost always engaged in for the *purpose of* something else. One says: 'I must get some sleep *in order that* I wake refreshed tomorrow.' 'I must go to bed *in order that* I work effectively …' and so on. This suggests that sleep is almost always purposeful, and tied, in a way, to all of our other ends—our life projects. So our choosing with regard to sleep, for instance, isn't really choosing sleep at all. It's choosing the parameters of our sleep time, always with our purposes in mind.

Chapter 12

Categories of Constraint and Avenues of Freedom: Proposing Collective Agency for Addressing Problems of Obesity

Catherine A. Womack
Bridgewater State College, USA

Obesity and Agency

Obesity is a problem of epidemic proportions, affecting both developed and developing countries. The spread of technology, the rise of global commerce, the changing nature of work and shifts in family social roles are among the factors blamed for changing the food supply and daily activities of people all over the world. In the United States, one of the fattest countries in the world, an estimated 66 per cent of its residents are overweight, and of those, about 32 per cent are obese.[1] Most health experts also blame the problem on sedentary lifestyles and diets that include mostly energy-dense (high-fat, high-sugar, high-calorie) food. In short, we eat too much and don't exercise enough.

This seems like a simple problem. If excess calorie intake is the problem, then we should simply reduce the number of calories we consume and burn more of them. In short, we should eat less and exercise more. Plans offering ways to adjust our daily diet by restricting or eliminating certain foods abound; however, these regimens are hard to follow, and lifestyle changes are even harder to maintain over the long term.

Why should some extra poundage among the citizenry be a source of worry? For one thing, there are many studies linking obesity to increased risk for type-II diabetes, heart disease, some cancers, arthritis and other health problems.[2] There is also a dimension to the obesity problem that merits philosophical investigation.

---

[1] For extensive data on obesity rates in the US, see the National Center for Health Statistics website: http://www.cdc.gov/nchs/products/pubs/pubd/hestats/overwght99.htm#Table%201 (accessed July 2007).

[2] For one of many sites with information about health risks associated with obesity, see: http://www.surgeongeneral.gov/topics/obesity/calltoaction/fact_consequences.htm (accessed July 2007).

Dieting is ubiquitous, but if studies are to be believed, it is completely ineffective for weight loss. People cannot seem to effect long-term dietary changes. This happens despite the prevalence of strong anti-fat prejudices; a 1988 study found that students would prefer to marry an embezzler, a cocaine user, a shoplifter or a blind person rather than an obese person.[3] If individual control over body weight is limited, then to address problems of obesity effectively, individual programmes are not a solution. It is precisely this line of reasoning I will use in this article.

Obesity is a medical, public health, public policy, economic, and social problem. It also presents philosophical problems to be solved: problems about causation, choice and human agency. I will use obesity as a lens through which to examine questions of choice and agency. In particular, given a multiplicity of constraints on our abilities to engage in certain types of eating and activity behaviours, how can we find avenues of freedom for choice and pathways to real agency for ourselves and our communities? I will examine some ways in which individuals are limited with respect to control over eating, and then propose some avenues for collective agency through changing our eating infrastructures.

Causes of Obesity: A Heterogeneous Landscape

Unravelling the causes of obesity is complicated because there are so many factors playing a role in determining body weight. These factors range from features of our genetics to broad characteristics of our cultures. Research on connections between human genetics and body weight variation is vigorous and ongoing; many published papers speculate (based on preliminary empirical data) on the causal roles of various genetic markers and their roles in weight regulation. However, there is significant agreement that genetics contributes strongly to one's body weight.[4] How strongly and in what ways (e.g. through variation in hunger/satiety patterns, efficiency and location of fat storage, etc.) are still issues yet to be settled.[5]

Social scientists are investigating socioeconomic determinants of obesity, revealing connections with race, gender, ethnicity, culture income, and marital

---

[3] M. Tiggeman and E.D. Rothblum, 'Gender Differences in Social Consequences of Perceived Overweight in the United States and Australia', *Sex Roles*, 18 (1988): 75-86.

[4] There are hundreds of studies investigating these connections. See, for instance: H. Hermine, M. Maes, M.C. Neale and L.J. Eaves, 'Genetic and Environmental Factors in Relative Body Weight and Human Adiposity', *Behavior Genetics*, 27/4 (1997); S. O'Rahilly and I.S. Farooqi, 'Genetics of Obesity', *Philosophical Transactions of the Royal Society of London, Biological Sciences*, 29/361 (1471) (2006): 1095-105.

[5] For good non-technical treatments on both the background and future directions of research on genetics and obesity, see E.R. Shell, *The Hungry Gene: The Science of Fat and the Future of Thin* (New York: Atlantic Monthly Press, 2002); see also R. Pool, *Fat: Fighting the Obesity Epidemic* (New York: Oxford University Press, 2001).

status. The Boston-based hunger advocacy agency 'Project Bread' published a report citing many connections between hunger and obesity.[6] For instance, children in low-income families often lack safe places to play outside, and are less likely to engage in organized physical activity. Access to supermarkets is also limited or nonexistent in poor neighbourhoods. Also, some studies have shown that women who cannot afford nutritionally adequate food are more likely to be obese than those who can. These results and others suggest multiple socioeconomic causal determinants of obesity.

Harvard Law professor Jon Hanson and colleagues have done extensive analysis on how corporations, through advertising and marketing, profoundly influence consumers' eating behaviours.[7] Their conclusions rest on a two-pronged argument. First, they cite the large body of evidence from social psychology, including the infamous Milgram[8] experiments, that strongly suggests that individual human behaviours are not the result of individual beliefs and desires; rather, people are highly susceptible to situational influences from external features of their environments.

In the second prong of the argument, Hanson et al. argue that commercial interests work to direct potential customers to buy their products by first manipulating them through the use of external eating cues in advertising, and then reframing the advertising campaigns and resulting behaviours (e.g. buying and consuming products) in terms of consumer choice. By emphasizing individual responsibility, Hanson claims that corporations can avoid, among other things, federal regulation of food advertising, particularly advertising aimed at children.

The Institute of Medicine, in a study on the causes of childhood obesity, concurs with Hanson about the effects of food advertising[9] on obesity. Food advertising and marketing targeted at children are cited as a main contributing factor, and the authors argue for development of food industry guidelines or, in their absence, government regulation.

---

[6] Supporting studies can be found in a publication by Project Bread, 'The Link Between Hunger and Obesity': http://www.projectbread.org/site/DocServer/TheLinkBetweenHungerAndObesity_2004.pdf?docID=104 (accessed July 2007)

[7] See especially A. Benforado, J. Hanson and D. Yosifon 'Broken Scales: Obesity and Justice in America', *Emory Law Review*, 53 (2004): 1645.

[8] The literature on and by Milgram is vast; one of his most influential early works is *Obedience to Authority: An Experimental View* (New York: Harper & Row, 1974).

[9] For a comprehensive analysis of causes of childhood obesity as well as policy recommendations, see Institute of Medicine (US) Committee on Prevention of Obesity in Children and Youth, *Preventing Childhood Obesity: Health in the Balance*, (eds) C.T. Liverman, V.I. Kraak, J.P. Koplan (Washington, DC: National Academies Press, 2005).

Focus on Dieting: A Dire Prognosis

Even though there are many disparate causes of obesity, medical science has, for the most part, settled on individual behaviours as where the most important causes lie. Let us look briefly at the effectiveness of dieting on long-term weight loss and maintenance. Then, we will examine what assumptions underlie the emphasis on dieting as an approach to addressing obesity.

In order to be effective, it seems reasonable that a diet meet the following criteria: it should result in adequate weight loss, help people keep weight off in the long term and be feasible to follow and maintain. Let us examine each in turn.

In a recent study comparing one-year weight losses for Atkins, Ornish, Zone and Weight Watcher diets, researchers found no significant differences between the groups, and only modest (5-8 pounds) average weight losses after one year.[10] Another study, comparing weight loss among groups of obese subjects divided into different weight loss programmes, found that, after very modest weight loss (no greater than 9.5 pounds on average), losses at the two-year mark ranged from 6.4 pounds to .5 pounds.[11] Many other studies corroborate these findings; for any medical diet regimen, even accompanied with behaviour modification and activity plans, weight losses are generally small (no more than 5 per cent of body weight), and over the long term, most subjects regain much of what they originally lost.

To measure feasibility of a diet, researchers tend to look at compliance rates; that is, what percentage of experimental subjects completes the study. In general, compliance rates are relatively low; less than 60 per cent on average. Outside of the lab, anecdotal reports of difficulties adhering to diets are commonplace. In short, diets do not seem to be an effective means of weight loss and maintenance. Why not? We will address this question in the following section.

Signs of the Need for a Conceptual Shift on Obesity

There is a strong presumption that the solution for regulation of body weight lies in finding the right combination of food intake/activity. According to this view, what people need in order to lose weight is expert information about the optimal food/activity plan, as well as sufficient motivation and a sense of personal responsibility, which are the keys to weight maintenance. What is wrong with this picture?

With respect to the former, there is good reason to believe that there is no single optimal food/activity plan for weight loss and maintenance. First, there is no consensus among medical experts on diet and nutrition about which combinations and amounts

---

[10] Dansinger, et al., 'Comparison of the Atkins, Ornish, Weight Watchers, and Zone Diets for Weight Loss and Heart Disease Risk Reduction: A Randomized Trial', *JAMA*, 293 (2005): 43-53.

[11] The Council on Size and Weight Discrimination. 'Long Term Diet Failure': http://www.cswd.org/docs/ltdietstudy.html (accessed July 2007).

of foods comprise an effective weight loss or maintenance plan. There are basic disagreements, for example, over what percentage of carbohydrates or fats should be included in a food plan, and what short and long-term effects are brought about by altering these percentages.[12] There are also disagreements about the possibility of food addiction patterns; one debate concerns the extent to which ingestion of sugar causes an addiction-response in the brain.[13] The answer to this research question will have strong ramifications for any medically-prescribed diet plan.

Another sort of evidence is found among a small group of diet success stories. The National Weight Control Registry[14] tracks individuals in a database of more than 5,000 people who have lost at least 30 pounds and kept it off for at least a year. Researchers searched to find common patterns for successful weight loss and, more importantly, successful long-term weight maintenance. It turns out that successful long-term weight maintainers:[15] (1) get enough sleep; (2) eat breakfast; (3) tend to eat lower fat meals (<25 per cent); (4) weigh themselves regularly; (5) eat consistently throughout the week (no bingeing); and (6) engage in regular and often vigorous exercise.

However, researchers could find that no one particular diet regimen dominated the group. Some eat low-carb, some eat low-fat, some engage in more calorie restriction, some eat less varied diets; all this suggests that there is no magic formula for dieting one's way to a long-term stable weight. On the brighter side, this evidence suggests that there are instead multiple dietary paths to a healthy weight.

Let us turn to the second requirement for successful dieting: motivation and personal responsibility on the part of the dieter to implement a diet plan successfully over time.

As fodder for motivation, the medical effects of obesity are well-publicized to the general public. In addition to official government, academic and non-profit organizational sources,[16] popular magazine cover stories on the so-called obesity epidemic warn of connections between obesity and cancer, type-II diabetes,

---

[12] An informal survey of the range of diet books in any bookstore reveals wide variation in expert recommendations on quantity of food, variety, fat/carb/protein ratios, and frequency and size of meals, for instance.

[13] There is a large literature on this subject; an interesting online source with selected references is found on the Rudd Center for Food Policy and Obesity website at Yale University: http://www.yaleruddcenter.org/default.aspx?id=68

[14] Their website, containing research results, anecdotal stories, and information for those interested in joining the registry, is: http://www.nwcr.ws/

[15] A bibliography of research papers with these findings can be found at: http://www.nwcr.ws/Research/default.htm

[16] For instance, see the Weight Control Information Network, part of the National Institute of Diabetes and Digestive and Kidney Diseases (NIDDK): http://win.niddk.nih.gov/statistics/index.htm. See also NAASO, The Obesity Society: http://www.naaso.org/statistics/obesity_trends.asp

and heart disease.[17] Popular culture has adopted obesity as a current concern; from television shows and magazines devoted to tips for successful weight loss to the mass marketing of diet programmes and products, consumers are deluged with information about weight, dieting and exercise, and the dangers of staying overweight or obese.

There is also ample motivation to be found in the pervasive anti-fat bias in many Western societies; there is a strong social stigma against being obese. In many studies conducted over the last few decades, everyone from schoolchildren to healthcare providers reported negative attitudes and behaviours towards the obese. One recent publication states that '28 per cent of teachers in one study said that becoming obese is the worst thing that can happen to a person; 24 per cent of nurses said that they are "repulsed" by obese persons; and, controlling for income and grades, parents provide less college support for their overweight than for their thin children.'[18]

Discrimination and bias against obesity even includes the obese themselves;[19] negative attitudes towards self and other obese people seem to be commonplace. However, unlike the case of smoking, stigmatizing a condition has not reduced its prevalence. According to a recent *New York Times* article,[20] researchers identified a counterintuitive consequence of stigmatizing obesity: it apparently makes the obese eat more. Since obese people participate in the same social norms of stigmatization as the rest of the population, it would stand to reason that if reversing the eating/activity patterns producing obesity were within one's power, one would certainly do so. But that has not happened. This suggests that the third element of the individualized solution for weight management personal responsibility is ill-placed.

Constraints and Complexities Surrounding Eating Choices

A series of studies with some surprising results done by Cornell's Brian Wansink[21] shows that external environmental cues can have a decided effect on our eating patterns in a variety of contexts.

---

17 For examples, see 'The Heavy Cost of Fat', *National Geographic* (August 2004) and 'Overcoming Obesity in America', *Time* (7 June 2004).

18 R. Puhl and K.D. Brownell, 'Bias, Discrimination, and Obesity', *Obesity Research*, 9 (2001): 788-805.

19 S.S. Wang, K.D. Brownell and T.A. Wadden, 'The Influence of the Stigma of Obesity on Overweight Individuals', *International Journal of Obesity*, 28 (2004): 1333-7.

20 G. Kolata, 'For a World of Woes, We Blame Cookie Monsters', New York Times (29 October 2006).

21 B. Wansink and SeaBum Park, 'At the Movies: How External Cues and Perceived Taste Impact Consumption Volume', *Food Quality and Preference*, 12/1 (January 2001): 69-74.

Food researchers have long believed that food consumption rates are in part a function of perceived food taste; in short, we eat more of what tastes good to us.[22] However, Wansink et al. argue that even with perceived lowered food quality, external features like container size are shown to influence people's eating behaviours. They conducted a test in which they gave moviegoers free popcorn in either a medium (120g) or large (240g) container, along with soda. After the movie, the subject filled out a short survey, giving information about a number of factors, including how much they liked the taste of the popcorn. Among the group who had a favourable view of the popcorn taste, the ones with larger containers ate 49 per cent more; oddly, in the group with an unfavourable taste view, those with the larger container ate 61 per cent more. One notable feature of this study: the researchers used ten-day-old popcorn for the subjects to consume. The researchers acknowledge that many factors account for the consumption increase, including mood and attention to eating. However, even in the absence of tasty food, people will overeat in response to external cues like larger container size.

Wansink conducted many similar studies to show the effects of environmental factors on eating patterns. Two studies showed that both children and adults pour and consume more juice when given a short, wide glass compared to those given a tall, narrow glass, but they perceive the opposite to be true.[23] The subjects given short, wide glasses poured 76 per cent more juice than those with the tall, narrow glasses. Furthermore, those with the short glasses thought they were consuming less juice. In other studies on visibility and placement of food in households and offices, they found that subjects eat more of foods within easy reach (e.g. chocolate kisses in a bowl on one's desk) and also more of a food if it is in a larger container (e.g. eating *M&Ms* from a two-pound bag vs. a half-pound bag). Wansink offers an explanation and suggests a strategy for dealing with this phenomenon: 'It appears that people use their eyes to count calories and not their stomachs. The importance of having salient, accurate visual cues can play an important role in the prevention of unintentional overeating.'[24]

There is a large body of research devoted to identifying what sorts of environmental cues are salient, and how they influence eating behaviours. The work of nutrition scientist Barbara Rolls[25] has examined in detail how portion size, volume, energy density (how high-calorie a food is), fat content, sugar content, accompanying liquid intake and other features affects how much we eat.

---

22 E.M. Bobroff and H.R. Kissileff, 'Effects of Changes in Palatability on Food Intake and the Cumulative Food Intake Curve in Man', *Appetite*, 7 (1986): 85-96.

23 B. Wansink and C. van Ittersum, 'Bottoms Up! The Influence of Elongation and Pouring on Consumption Volume', *Journal of Consumer Research*, 30/3 (2003): 455-63.

24 B. Wansink, J.E. Painter and J. North, 'Bottomless Bowls: Why Visual Cues of Portion Size May Influence Intake', *Obesity Research*, 13/1 (2005): 93-100.

25 For a list of Rolls' publications and those of her colleagues at the Penn State Laboratory for the Study of Human Ingestive Behavior, go to: http://nutrition.hhdev.psu.edu/foodlab/pubs/index.html (accessed July 2007).

In one study, Rolls et al. tested how adults responded to meals on different days of four different portion sizes of macaroni and cheese. They found that the subjects consumed 30 per cent more (162 calories) when offered the largest portion (1,000g) compared to the smallest portion (500g). They also reported similar ratings of hunger and fullness after each meal despite the intake differences. However, only 45 per cent of the subjects reported noticing the differences in the size of the portions served. In a different study, the researchers gave the same subjects different size sandwiches on different days to test the effects of increasing the portion size of a food served as a discrete unit. Men and women who were offered different size (6-, 8-, 10-, and 12inch) sub sandwiches for lunch on four different days ate significantly more as the size of the sandwich offered became larger.[26]

There are some key insights to be found in this type of research. First, in many food decision contexts, our calculations and conclusions are highly fallible. In many everyday contexts, we systematically misjudge volume, calorie content, nutritional quality and total amounts consumed of the foods we eat. Furthermore, the judgements made and beliefs used to embark on a course of action (e.g. eating a certain amount of soup) are based on tacit information; we do not have cognitive access to them. That is, we are not aware that proximity triggers us to eat more in the absence of hunger or desirability of food; we simply respond and act on that trigger. Also, human perceptual judgements about volume are flawed in ways known to researchers, but not to individuals; we can't see that we tend to underestimate volume in short, wide vessels even if we look carefully. We can come to learn about our limitations and implement strategies based on this acquired knowledge, but we must rely on research, not our own capacities, for the information.

These insights help dispel two myths about individual control over eating: first, explaining our eating behaviours is almost entirely determined by our beliefs, preferences and reasoning involving them; and second, that our bodies will send us clear signals about how much to eat and when we should stop; all we have to do is pay attention to and heed the signals. With respect to the latter, research has shown that many external cues trigger eating behaviours, even when we know what those cues are. And furthermore, those external cues seem to override or block whatever

---

[26] This research summary is taken from a Centers for Disease Control Research to Practice series on weight control and management; for more examples and an extensive bibliography, go to: http://www.cdc.gov/nccdphp/dnpa/nutrition/pdf/portion_size_research.pdf (accessed July 2007).

signals of satiety our bodies may be sending.[27] In an interview,[28] Wansink recounts his experience of giving a detailed 90-minute lecture to graduate students about external cues and eating behaviors. Six weeks later, he invited those students to a *Super Bowl* football party, where there were big bowls and small bowls of snack food. Despite their detailed knowledge about external eating cues, the students who ate from the large bowls nonetheless ate much more than those who ate from the small bowls, and underestimated how much they ate.

As for the former, our beliefs about important and basic features of food, like how much is before us, are clearly unreliable under certain circumstances, as the research results demonstrate. So, our perceptual and calculating abilities result in flawed decisions about how much to eat, thwarting genuine desires to eat moderately, healthily or comfortably. Even worse, the flawed information on which we base our decisions about eating is not even available for scrutiny or correction; we do not have cognitive access to the flawed rules until they are revealed by researchers. And, even when we have access to the relevant information, we still find it hard to act appropriately.

The Centers for Disease Control (CDC) offer advice for healthcare providers trying to help people lose weight and maintain it over time; they stress the importance of raising awareness about 'portion distortion', helping people assess what is the right amount to eat and teaching them how to control their food environments.[29] These approaches reflect the individualistic presuppositions about control and agency that pervade medical and even many public health views about weight control and management. Awareness of built-in human frailties surrounding food portions has been demonstrated to be ineffective in real-life contexts where external eating cues are strong (as in the *Super Bowl* party experiment by Wansink). Judging how much to eat may require a food scale, says the CDC, which is impractical in public eating situations; without it, people have trouble identifying reasonable portions of foods.

The above-mentioned research also suggests that we are strongly influenced by social conventions governing behaviours in cultural contexts like eating at parties, eating in restaurants, even eating commercially-prepared sandwiches.

---

27 Research on how satiety gets signalled and transmitted is ongoing; the point is that external features of our environments interfere with the ability to stop eating once a satiety-producing amount of food is consumed. How satiety mechanisms work and how exactly their messages get overridden, ignored, or overwritten is an important area for further investigation, but I would argue that such knowledge is not required in order to address the external cue problem of overeating.

28 Interview on Mindless Eating, *Here and Now* radio show, WBUR Boston, (Tuesday 21 November 2006). A recording of the interview is available at: http://www.here-now.org/shows/2006/11/20061121.asp (accessed July 2007).

29 For more details, see: http://www.cdc.gov/nccdphp/dnpa/nutrition/pdf/portion_size_research.pdf (accessed July 2007).

Exercising individual control in one of these contexts does not usually happen, even when we know that we are prone to overeating in precisely those contexts.

However, these revelations point to ways to take advantage of how we perceive and judge food and the various contexts of eating; we can use this information to exercise real control and real agency, resulting in satisfaction of individual needs and goals surrounding weight loss and management. In the final section, I will outline some modest proposals for collective approaches to addressing problems of obesity.

Finding Agency Within a Network of Constraints: Some Modest Proposals

We have seen that standard approaches to weight control focus on education and motivation for individual dieters, in the hope of effecting long-term sustainable behaviour change. Those approaches fail in the vast majority of cases, not because people lack information or will, but because the kinds of behaviours called for in the programmes are not those that people have control over. Educating dieters about appropriate portion sizes (e.g. 'the right amount of chicken for a meal is the size of a deck of cards') does not translate into eating less in many conventional contexts. Restaurant portions in the US are several times larger than the recommended amounts, and research has shown that people commonly misjudge the amount of food they are eating. Also, we cannot rely on signals of fullness to help us stop eating in many contexts; for whatever reason, the presence of some portion of food overrides those messages of satiety, leading to overeating.

So, if our perceptual and cognitive faculties often do not help us regulate eating, what can we do? Wansink suggests that research on external eating cues can be used to change the way, say, that food is packaged. Food that is already portion-controlled through division into smaller pre-packaged amounts is easier to eat in reasonable amounts. The food industry is already moving in this direction, marketing some snack foods in 100-calorie bags. Lobbying for more of this sort of packaging, with calorie amounts clearly labelled may help consumers eat in smaller amounts.

This example raises a general problem; there are many external tacit eating cues that we act on without our knowledge. Identifying them and forming strategies that do not require heroic (and futile) efforts by the individual, but rather changes in the food environment, seem promising. For instance, promoting size reduction in chain restaurants, fast-food venues and manufactured snack food may help reduce consumption. Other sorts of interventions will depend on what research on external cues reveals. Food advertising has already been shown to have effects on children. A more minute analysis of what sorts of cues are at work can help with efforts to regulate its influence.

Recognizing our cognitive, perceptual and social limitations is a first step towards finding pathways of real agency in our relationship with food. I have argued here that whereas we lack individual control in some contexts, we have access to second-order strategies that will make our eating environment one that allows us to choose what foods we want; at the same time, these strategies can help us achieve long-term goals of health and satisfaction. Research that focuses on features of the social structures in the community, rather than merely those of the individual, can better promote the general good of its members.

Chapter 13

Equipoise in Public Health Research

Marcel Verweij
Utrecht University, Netherlands

Introduction

A common scheme for childhood vaccinations is to vaccinate newborns three times during their first months, with a booster after a year. Such a 4-dose (3+1) scheme is standard in immunization programmes in most high-income countries, for vaccines against diphtheria, tetanus, poliomyelitis, and hepatitis B. The immune system of a very young child (<1 year) is only developing and therefore single infections or vaccinations may not cause a sufficient immune response at that time. Therefore, during the first month after birth, multiple vaccinations may be required in order to protect the child throughout its first year. After this period, sometimes a single vaccination may already offer sufficient protection for a number of years, as is the case with vaccines against measles and meningitis C.

Given that 3+1 is a more or less standard scheme for newborn immunizations, new vaccines are often tested using a similar schedule. For the sake of registration, pharmaceutical companies will tend to take a conservative approach to testing new vaccines; i.e. they will test new vaccines in a dose and schedule that is expected to show a clear effect. However, it is not clear *a priori* whether giving fewer vaccinations would be really insufficient. As soon as a vaccine is registered according to a 3+1 schedule, and even more when such a schedule is adopted in a national vaccination programme, it will be difficult to find out if a simpler scheme would be sufficiently effective as well. After all, if there is a proven effective method available, it will be controversial to study a different scheme, especially if such a test would involve placebo controls. Apart from that, pharmaceutical companies will have little reason to support research that may result in a reduction of vaccine sales.

On the other hand, governments or public health authorities may have several reasons for considering a reduced scheme. A reduced scheme will obviously be less expensive as it requires fewer injections and fewer doses of vaccine; as a result, it will also be less vulnerable to vaccine scarcities; and it leaves more room for further vaccinations against other diseases. And finally, whilst parents more often take a critical attitude towards vaccination, policies that explicitly adopt a 'no more vaccinations than strictly necessary' attitude may help to sustain public trust in childhood immunization programmes.

However, the possibility of reduced vaccination schemes raises ethical issues. If the effectiveness of a reduced scheme needs to be proven before it is accepted, can it be justified to test the reduced scheme against placebo? I will argue that such a trial does not satisfy the principle of equipoise. However, the main moral rationale of clinical equipoise, beneficence and the special duty of healthcare workers towards patients is not easily applicable to research in preventive medicine. Therefore, considerations of equipoise may be irrelevant in these cases. Another moral rationale for equipoise is the principle of fairness, and this can still be relevant, especially in circumstances where a reduced vaccination scheme would satisfy a clear public health need, as will often be the case in low-income countries.

This topic has clear parallels with the ongoing ethical debate about medical research in developing countries and critique of the *Declaration of Helsinki* which takes a very restrictive stance towards placebo-controlled trials. I will focus however on the moral rationale of equipoise, and only briefly reflect on requirements for placebo-controlled trials as such.

Vaccine trials raise numerous moral issues about safety, trust, exploitation, informed consent, and pre-randomization. In order to keep the focus on the topic of equipoise, I will simply assume in this paper that ethical requirements other than those related to equipoise are satisfied.

Although this analysis of research on reduced vaccination schemes is relevant for research on vaccination in general, and especially for developing world contexts, it will be helpful to start with a specific case in the Netherlands in which the problem of equipoise emerged.

Reduced Schemes for Pneumococcal Vaccination of Newborn Children

In 2002, the Health Council of the Netherlands recommended the government to adopt a new vaccine against pneumococcal disease in the national childhood vaccination programme.[1] The vaccine, when administered according to a 4-dose (3+1) scheme, had been proven effective in reducing a significant morbidity and mortality in young children. Pneumococcal infections can lead to serious, sometimes fatal disease, notably meningitis and sepsis. Children are especially vulnerable for pneumococcal disease in the first months after birth. Pneumococcal infections may also cause other, more common diseases during childhood, such as otitis media. The Health Council estimated that pneumococcal vaccinations at months 2, 3, and 4, and a booster after 12 months might prevent up to 100 cases of meningitis and sepsis, 3,200 cases of pneumonia, and tens of thousands of cases of otitis media. Approximately 10 per cent of the cases of pneumococcal meningitis

[1] Gezondheidsraad, *Algemene Vaccinatie tegen Meningokokken C en* Pneumokokken [Health Council of Netherlands (2002) Universal Vaccination Against Meningococcal Serogroup C and Pneumococcal Disease.] (Den Haag: Gezondheidsraad, 2002.)

and sepsis would have been fatal, and another 10 per cent would have resulted in lifelong health problems.[2] The pneumococcal vaccine is however also expensive, and the Health Council estimated that the costs per Quality Adjusted Life Year gained would be high in comparison to other prevention programmes. As a result the Minister of Health decided to postpone the introduction of this vaccine.

In the USA, the Centers for Disease Control (CDC) also recommended vaccinating children according to a 4-dose (3+1) schedule. In 2004 however, vaccine-scarcity necessitated the CDC to suspend the fourth and later also the third dose of pneumococcal vaccine.[3] It appeared that even with two injections in the first months after birth, a vaccine effectiveness of 94 per cent was realized. Some other immunological studies also support the hypothesis that a reduced scheme would offer a level of protection that is similar to the standard 4-dose scheme.[4]

In the Netherlands this led to questions whether introducing a 3-dose (months 2, 4 and 12) vaccination could offer sufficient protection for children and be affordable for government. In a follow-up report, the Health Council argued that there was as yet inadequate clinical evidence for such a decision.[5] A scientifically-warranted decision about a 3-dose schedule would require either a comparative equivalence study (3-dose versus 4-dose), or a trial in which a 3-dose scheme was tested against placebo. Of these options, the placebo-controlled trial would be most feasible: a head-to-head comparison of the 3-dose and the 4-dose scheme would require much more time and more (probably far too many) participants.[6] Yet a placebo-controlled study might be morally problematic given that the vaccine (in a 4-dose schedule) had already been proven effective.

---

[2] Ibid., p. 23.

[3] Centers for Disease Control, 'Updated Recommendations on the Use of Pneumococcal Conjugate Vaccine: Suspension of Recommendation for Third and Fourth Dose', *Morbidity and Mortality Weekly Report*, 53/8 (2004): 177-8.

[4] D. Goldblatt and J. Southern, et al., 'Immunogenicity and Boosting After a Reduced Number of Doses of a Pneumococcal Conjugate Vaccine in Infants and Toddlers', *Pediatric Infectious Disease Journal*, 25/4 (2006): 312-19.

[5] Gezondheidsraad, *Vaccinatie van Zuigelingen tegen Pneumokokkeninfecties [Vaccination of Infants Against Pneumococcal Disease]* (Den Haag: Gezondheidsraad, 2005).

[6] This is a controversial issue. In general equivalency studies may not require a much larger sample size then placebo-controlled studies. See B. Freedman, C. Weijer, and K.C. Glass, 'Placebo Orthodoxy in Clinical research. I: Empirical and Methodological Myths', *Journal of Law Medicine and Ethics*, 24 (1996): 243-51. Equivalency studies are in a way simpler as they only need to show that certain interventions satisfy a pre-established level of efficacy, and this has implications for the number of subjects required. In this paper I will however assume that choosing a placebo-controlled trial does make sense from a methodological point of view, in order to examine whether it can be morally justified, given lack of equipoise. Even if an equivalency trial would be feasible in a case like this, whether it is morally preferable to a placebo-controlled trial will depend on the arguments I will discuss.

In the end, the discussion about introducing a 3-dose schedule was set aside. An update of cost-effectiveness data of a 4-dose scheme led to the conclusion that such a policy was less expensive then previously assumed, and the Dutch government decided to introduce a 4-dose pneumococcal vaccination in the childhood vaccination programme after all.

This decision however does not render the question about placebo-controlled studies with a proven effective vaccine irrelevant. After all, if a reduced (3-dose) vaccination schedule would offer sufficient protection, then the marginal benefits of a fourth vaccine might not justify the inconveniences. Moreover, opting for a reduced dose would create room for other vaccines, and it might reinforce public trust in the programme.

Equipoise and 'Treating the Best One Can'

One problem that is raised if a reduced vaccination scheme is tested against a placebo is that such a study will not satisfy the principle of equipoise. The concept of equipoise was first introduced by the philosopher Charles Fried, who had concerns about the morality of randomized clinical trials.[7] The principle of equipoise holds that it is immoral for a physician to enrol patients in a trial in which two treatments are compared, if the physician has a clear medical preference for one treatment over the other. Randomization can only be justified if the physician is in a state of equipoise, that is, if she is genuinely uncertain which of the treatments is the better one. In other words, she should have an honest null-hypothesis. Equipoise can be considered as a medical-ethical requirement that flows from the principle of beneficence and the special commitments a physician has towards her patients. The fiduciary relationship between physician and patient implies that the physician has a commitment to care for her patient the best she can.[8] Randomizing patients in a trial where there is no equipoise is wrong because it would imply that the physician is offering some patients inferior treatment, and that is something she cannot reasonably justify to those patients. From a moral point of view, such randomization is not in the best interests of the patient, and hence the physician does not satisfy her professional duty. From a legal point of view, offering inferior treatment can be considered as negligence.

The concept of equipoise has been developed by Benjamin Freedman, who argues that equipoise should not refer to the beliefs and preferences of an individual physician or researcher but to the opinion of the wider medical community.[9]

---

7 C. Fried, *Medical Experimentation: Personal Integrity and Social Policy* (Amsterdam: Elsevier, 1974).

8 P.B. Miller and C. Weijer, 'Rehabilitating Equipoise', *Kennedy Institute of Ethics Journal*, 13/2 (2003): 93-118.

9 B. Freedman, 'Equipoise and the Ethics of Clinical Research', *New England Journal of Medicine*, 317 (1987): 141-5.

Clinical equipoise requires that there is genuine uncertainty within the expert community about the treatments that are compared. If some clinicians involved in the trial think that treatment A will be better than treatment B, this is not yet sufficient for the trial to be unacceptable. As long as there is disagreement within the larger expert community about which is best, testing A against B does not violate the principle of equipoise.

What does the principle imply for research in which a reduced vaccination scheme is tested against placebo? Let us focus on the example of pneumococcal vaccination. A series of four vaccinations (months 2, 3, 4 and 12) has been proven safe and it has been shown effective in raising antibody response and preventing pneumococcal disease in children. It is reasonable to assume that a reduced vaccination scheme (months 2, 4, and 12) will be at least as safe as the accepted scheme, and that it will have a protective effect. The effect level might be somewhat lower than the 4-dose scheme, but there must be a clear difference between a 3-dose vaccination schedule and placebo. Though there may have been no appropriate clinical studies that establish the effects of a 3-dose scheme, there will be sufficient evidence that even a single dose of vaccine will produce immune responses that protect against infections with the targeted micro-organism. It is not clear how strong this protective effect will be and how long it will last in children during their first year. The effect curves of the various treatments (placebo, 3-dose and 4-dose) over time could be something like in the graph below. The graph illustrates how 4-dose vaccine will offer a very high level of protection starting at the first injection. The lower curve refers to some effect a placebo might have. The middle curve of a 3-dose vaccination scheme illustrates how such a scheme may offer a lower level of protection, especially between months 6-12. After a booster vaccination at 12 months, however, children may be expected to be as well-protected as in a full vaccination schedule.

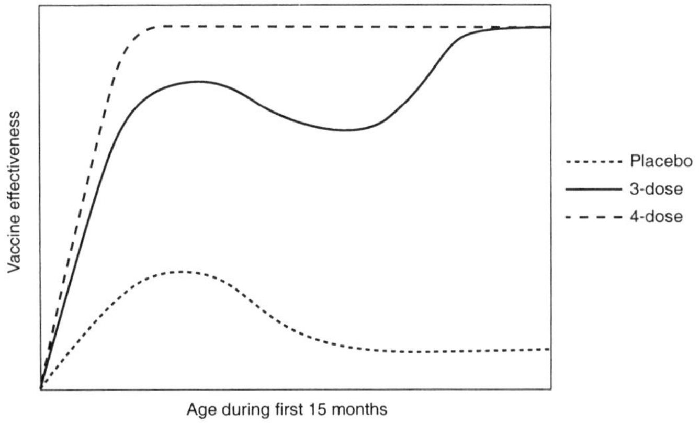

Figure 13.1 Relative Effectiveness of Placebo, 4-Dose Schedule, 3-Dose Schedule

Now a placebo-controlled trial is proposed to study the clinical effectiveness of a 3-dose pneumococcal vaccination scheme. It seems clear that such a trial does not satisfy the principle of equipoise. Given the available knowledge about the effectiveness and safety of the vaccine, I assume that it is beyond doubt that even a reduced scheme of vaccination will offer a level of protection that goes beyond the effect of a placebo. From a medical perspective, vaccination (even in a reduced scheme) is preferable to placebo, and hence there is no equipoise between both arms of the study. Of course, there is uncertainty about how effective the reduced scheme is, hence how much the middle curve differs from the lower curve—that is the reason for proposing a study like this. If equipoise is required for clinical trials, then this proposed study cannot be acceptable from a moral point of view. However, is this conclusion as straightforward as it seems?

The Limited Relevance of Equipoise in Prevention Research

First of all, it is not obvious that the moral rationale for equipoise applies to vaccine trials with healthy subjects in a similar way as it does to other clinical trials. As explained above, the moral requirement of equipoise flows from the commitment of a physician to her patients. A physician should treat her patients the best she can. In a trial where the arms are not in equipoise, some subjects get a treatment that, from a medical perspective, is inferior. This is something a physician cannot justify to patients who are ill and need treatment in order to regain health, or for relief of their symptoms, especially not if the superior treatment is readily available. In such a case the inferior treatment cannot be in the best interest of the patient, and the physician is morally obliged to offer the superior treatment.

However, the case at hand is a trial in which a preventive intervention is tested. The projected research subjects are healthy and not in need of specific medical treatment. We still assume that for them, given the risks of pneumococcal disease, receiving a vaccine is better than receiving a placebo. Yet, unless this specific vaccination is already standard practice, it is not obvious that physicians or public health nurses have a moral obligation to give the vaccine, and that for that reason giving a placebo would be wrong. Pneumococcal vaccination is only one of numerous preventive interventions (including other vaccines) that may help to prevent disease in children, and children and their parents cannot reasonably require that public health physicians offer any preventive treatment that is expected to reduce risk within a population. Preventive treatment is often organized collectively, as a programme in which various interventions (for example, several vaccines) are combined.

Which treatments are offered, and which are not, is subject to political decision-making, which, ideally is well-informed by evidence from medicine and public health. Parents can reasonably expect public health practitioners to recommend and offer preventive care that is part of the standard package. From a legal point of view, this package determines what they are entitled to. If less is offered for no good reason, this may well be considered a case of negligence. Yet the package also sets limits as to how far a public health physician or nurse must go in acting 'in the best interests' of the child. Children are not legally entitled to receive potentially beneficial vaccines (or other preventive forms of care) that are not part of the collective programme. Moreover, if the standard immunization programme does contain vaccines that are most important, given existing public health risks, healthy children may benefit from further vaccinations, but they will not need them in any strict sense.

This discussion seems to render the principle of equipoise, as far as it is based upon special duties of beneficence that are essential to the fiduciary relationship between physician and patient, inapplicable to prevention trials with healthy research subjects. Unless the study treatment is part of the current standard of preventive care, physicians cannot be morally required to give the better treatment. The moral rationale for equipoise is most clear in cases where healthcare professionals have a moral commitment to give the treatment their patients need. In studies in preventive medicine, the principle of equipoise may not be applicable. A trial in which the preventive effects of two interventions are compared can be morally acceptable, even if there is no equipoise regarding these arms of the study.

Public Health Needs, Equipoise and Fairness

The conclusion of the previous section is however too hasty if it is not qualified in a number of ways. A central premise in the argument is that there is a collective immunization programme that specifies which vaccines a child is entitled to; and that public health physicians do not have an obligation to offer more than that. The unspoken assumption is that this collective programme does meet the basic public health needs of the population. However, in many countries, public health is far from ideal and possibilities for collective immunization may be limited. This creates a completely different context for the evaluation of equipoise in public health studies. Suppose a national collective immunization programme is very limited and does not meet the basic public health needs of the population. Several disabling infectious diseases are endemic, but a vaccine that is known to be effective is considered too expensive if administered in a 4-dose schedule. Now public health authorities propose to start a placebo-controlled trial to test the effectiveness of an affordable, reduced schedule. This trial would, I think, create grave moral problems for physicians who are responsible for preventive care in the population. Even though the target groups are healthy children, their conditions are of course, far from healthy. Several diseases are endemic which means that children run a significant risk of becoming infected and developing illness. It is not unreasonable to claim that children in such a context *need* vaccination, and this has moral implications for the relationship between healthcare workers and their 'clients'. This case is more similar to research with patients, who need treatment for their ailments, and, as I have argued, in such a context the moral rationale for the principle of equipoise is clear and relevant.

Can a physician in this context justify randomizing children over two arms of a study (placebo versus vaccination) if she knows that they all need the protection the vaccine can offer to some extent? Clearly, receiving the vaccine would be in the best interest of every child. At this point however, no child is legally entitled to get the vaccine, given that it is not yet made collectively available. Some may argue that these children do have a moral right to vaccination, yet such a right is rather impotent if there is no vaccine that can be administered. Hence, even the physician who is caring for the children the best she can, will not be able—hence cannot have a moral obligation—to offer vaccination. So, if the physician has moral reasons to resist co-operating in this placebo-controlled trial, these reasons cannot be based on her special duty of beneficence towards each child.

A more relevant reason for public health professionals and other physicians to resist this placebo-controlled trial is however one of *fairness*. If all children run a clear risk to get ill and therefore need protection against the disease, it is unfair to offer protection to only some and not all of them. The randomization schedule that allocates placebos and vaccines to children makes the whole programme even more unjust. This may seem odd if one considers randomization to be a fair procedure. How could it be unfair to use a fair procedure? However, allocating resources at random is not fair if there are good substantive reasons for priority-setting. In most cases, allocating benefits and burdens on the basis of a lottery would be clearly unjust (Olympic medals) or even horrible (famine relief). A lottery can only be a fair instrument for distributing important goods if all reasons for prioritizing one group over another are exactly in balance.[10] In this case, arguably some children are more vulnerable then others, and this may tip the balance of reasons to their benefit. Hence there may be good medical reasons for allocating scarce vaccines in a particular way, and therefore a responsible physician should not accept randomization. In contrast to our discussion in the previous section, the principle of equipoise is morally important in a case like this. The rationale however is not beneficence and professional commitment to a patient, but fairness.

Individual healthcare workers may consider this as a dilemma between fairness (not co-operating in the trial) and beneficence (vaccinating at least part of the target group) but this only shows that the basic moral problem exceeds their agency. The problem of fairness partly results from the fact that scarcity is artificial and avoidable: it is a consequence of the decision to start a placebo-controlled study. So far the assumption was that a collective programme with a reduced vaccination scheme would be affordable in this hypothetical country. Why not then start the programme without further ado? True, there is still uncertainty about how effective a reduced scheme would be, and whether the protective effect is more or less similar to the effect of a full vaccination schedule. However, in a context where a dangerous infectious disease is endemic, a vaccine that is,

10 J. Broome, 'Selecting People Randomly', *Ethics*, 95 (1984): 38-55.

say, only 50 per cent effective, could be a major improvement to public health. Given that the full vaccination scheme may not be affordable anyway, it is rather uninteresting to find out if a reduced schedule would indeed be almost as good as the full schedule. Public health authorities in a context like this have good reasons to implement vaccination according to a reduced scheme, and to forgo further (placebo-controlled) studies. In this way they also avoid moral dilemmas for public health professionals in practice.

Controversies Over Placebo-Controlled Trials With Less Expensive Treatment Regimens

Research projects that aim to study medical interventions that are less expensive and probably less effective than existing methods may not satisfy the principle of equipoise, especially if such trials involve placebo controls. Such projects are highly controversial, but especially from a public health perspective it makes sense to develop therapeutic and preventive measures that are less expensive than existing options, and which therefore may become available and create benefits for a much larger group of persons.[11]

The central claim in this paper is that, in *prevention* trials with healthy subjects, equipoise may be not as important as in therapeutic research with patients who need treatment. I have argued that there are two distinct moral reasons for rejecting non-equipoised trials: (a) healthcare professionals may have a special duty of beneficence to care for their patients or clients the best they can, and (b) it may be unfair to randomize persons who all need certain preventive or therapeutic care, so that some will get the care they need and others will not. The first reason will not apply in preventive medicine if the preferable treatment is not part of a collective standard or public health programme. The second reason will only apply in circumstances where basic public health needs are unmet.[12]

Placebo-controlled trials with reduced, less expensive treatment regimens have raised a lot of controversy since 1997, when Lurie and Wolfe criticized a large number of HIV studies in developing countries.[13] The debate has focused since

[11] D.R. Buchanan, and F.G. Miller, 'Justice and Fairness in the Kennedy Krieger Institute Lead Paint Study: the Ethics of Public Health Research on Less Expensive, Less Effective Interventions', *American Journal of Public Health*, 96/5 (2006): 781-7.

[12] For the example of pneumococcal vaccination in the Netherlands this implies that, at the time of the controversy, there were no compelling moral reasons against a 3-dose versus placebo trial. However, if parents do understand that a 3-dose vaccination will be preferable to a placebo, then many may object to participation, and this could have made the whole trial unfeasible after all.

[13] P. Lurie and S.M. Wolfe, 'Unethical Trials of Interventions to Reduce Perinatal Transmission of the Human Immunodeficiency Virus in Developing Countries', *New England Journal of Medicine*, 337/12 (1997): 853-6.

then on the *Declaration of Helsinki* which takes a restrictive stance towards the acceptability of placebo-controlled trials, and on different concepts of the 'standard of care' that should apply in research in developing countries.[14] According to the *Declaration of Helsinki*: 'The benefits, risks, burdens and effectiveness of a new method should be tested against those of the best current prophylactic, diagnostic, and therapeutic methods'. In a by now much discussed footnote, the Declaration makes room for placebo-controlled studies, even when a proven method exists, in case it is scientifically necessary to use placebo controls in order to test the efficacy or safety of a prophylactic, diagnostic, and therapeutic method. The other exception is research where 'patients who receive placebo will not be subject to any additional risk of serious or irreversible harm'. Obviously, the *Declaration of Helsinki* does not make a distinction between preventive and therapeutic research. However, I have argued that such a distinction may be relevant when analyzing equipoise and the justification of placebo-controls.

One reason why the distinction between preventive and therapeutic trials has been often overlooked in recent debates is that the projects criticized by Lurie and Wolfe are indeed studies in preventive medicine. The objective was to establish the effectiveness of various relatively inexpensive interventions to prevent perinatal HIV transmission. The fact that these were prevention trials however did not play a major role in the ethical debates over equipoise and placebo-controlled trials, probably because the primary research subjects, HIV-seropositive pregnant women, were also patients who needed therapeutic treatment which they obviously did not receive. I have argued that in such circumstances the moral rationale of the principle of equipoise is relevant.

---

[14] World Medical Assembly, *Declaration of Helsinki: Ethical Principles for Medical Research Involving Human Subjects* (Edinburgh, 2000). Several articles that offer a clear insight in the debate are: A.J. London, 'The Ambiguity and the Exigency: Clarifying "Standard of Care" Arguments in International Research', *Journal of Medicine and Philosophy*, 25/4 (2000): 379-97; J.R. McMillan and C. Conlon, 'The Ethics of Research Related to Health Care in Developing Countries', *Journal of Medical Ethics*, 30 (2004): 204-6; R.K. Lie, E. Emanuel, and D. Wendler, 'The Standard of Care Debate: the Declaration of Helsinki Versus the International Consensus Opinion', *Journal of Medical Ethics*, 30 (2004): 190-93; U. Schüklenk, 'The Standard of Care Debate: Against the Myth of an "International Consensus Opinion"', *Journal of Medical Ethics*, 30 (2004): 194-7.

Chapter 14
Closing the Book on Infectious Disease: The Mischievous Consequences for Bioethics and for Public Health

Leslie P. Francis, Margaret P. Battin, Jay A. Jacobson, and Charles B. Smith
University of Utah, USA

Public health is a field of longstanding origins.[1] From the construction of aqueducts and sewers in ancient Rome, to efforts to combat plague in medieval Europe, to the origins of the United States Public Health Service in the care of injured merchant seamen in 1798,[2] to Dr John Snow's famous attribution of cholera to London's Broad Street pump in 1854, efforts to improve population health have been a matter of public concern. Bioethics, by contrast, is a relative latecomer as a field, emerging during the period of the late 1950s through the 1970s. Ethical analysis in each of these fields, however, has been shaped by the optimism of the 1960s and 1970s—the immediate pre-HIV/AIDS period—that infectious disease had largely been conquered. In this paper, we explore the ethical significance of this omission of infectious disease, arguing that it contributed to an unfortunate separation between the early development of bioethics and the field of public health. The advent of HIV/AIDS, we argue, did little to bridge the gap; what were regarded as 'exceptional' features of HIV/AIDS truncated appreciation of the theoretical challenges infectious diseases poses more generally for public health and bioethics.

The formative time period of bioethics coincides with the era of civil rights activism and legal responses, from *Brown v. Board of Education of Topeka*[3] in 1954 to the *Civil Rights Act* of 1964 and the *Age Discrimination in Employment Act* of 1967. This was also a period of growing environmental concern, fuelled by the publication of Rachel Carson's *Silent Spring* in 1962[4] and implemented by the *National Environmental Policy Act* of 1964, the *Clean Air Act* of 1970, and the *Clean Water Act* of 1972. And it was a period, before the advent of HIV/

[1] This chapter is based on M.P. Battin, L.P. Francis, J.A. Jacobson, and C.B. Smith, *Bioethics and Infectious Disease: The Patient as Victim and Vector* (Oxford: Oxford University Press, 2008).

[2] http://www.usphs.gov/html/history.html (accessed January 2007).

[3] *Brown v. Board of Education of Topeka*, 347 US 483 (1954).

[4] R. Carson, *Silent Spring* (Boston: Houghton-Mifflin, 1962).

AIDS, when infectious disease was increasingly regarded as a receding problem, a health threat largely conquered. The pronouncement attributed to the United States Surgeon General, purportedly closing the book on infectious disease, reflected this optimism.[5] This optimism—in retrospect so obviously unwarranted—was simply assumed as the field of bioethics developed. Perhaps even more surprisingly, similar optimism was to be found to a certain extent in the field of public health as well; attention in public health during the same time period was increasingly devoted to environmental hazards and to patterns of problematic behaviour such as smoking or weight gain. Only with the emergence of HIV/AIDS—and then in the main focused only on HIV/AIDS—did characteristic features of infectious diseases return to the fore for discussion, and even then in a limited way.

The discipline of public health, to be sure, continued to consider the spread of disease and the overall health of the population. But in public health discussions, too, during the period of the early development of bioethics, attention had shifted away from infectious disease to problems such as the health effects of cigarettes or DDT and other environmental toxins.[6] Writers in public health, like writers in bioethics, viewed infectious disease as largely conquered; ethical problems like the protection of confidentiality were set aside as largely moot. Although the fields of public health and public health law featured discussions that recognized the differences between aggregative, population-based approaches and the individualism of clinical medicine, scholars in the field of bioethics and in the field of public health rarely engaged with each other in ways that brought their paradigms of analysis into fruitful dialogue. Quite recently, this has begun to change, as the American Public Health Association has published a code of ethics (in 2002)[7] and a number of special issues of journals in bioethics have been devoted to the ethics of public health or to ethical issues that are highly salient to the field of public health, such as international human rights and health. Nonetheless, until quite recently, we argue here, the public health discussions and the field of bioethics developed separately, and the twain never really met.

These formative developments—the absence of attention to infectious disease in early bioethics, and the failure of extensive dialogue between public health

[5] The statement that 'it is time to close the book on infectious disease' was reportedly made by then Surgeon General William Stewart in testimony before Congress. We have been unable to locate an original source for the statement, although there are many secondary references.

[6] See, e.g., Carson, *Silent Spring*. The term 'bioethics' actually originated in discussions of ethics and the biosphere, but quickly came to be applied to ethical issues in healthcare. It is interesting to speculate whether links between bioethics and public health might have been forged much earlier, had 'bioethics' continued to encompass not only human but also environmental health. See, e.g., P.J. Whitehouse, 'The Rebirth of Bioethics: Extending the Original Formulations of Van Rensselaer Potter', *American Journal of Bioethics*, 3/4 (2003): W21-6.

[7] See http://www.apha.org/codeofethics/ethics.htm (accessed June 2006).

and the new field of bioethics—were not benign. The virtual omission of issues concerning infectious disease and the lack of awareness of the characteristic features of infectious disease affected the choice, framing, and discussion of problems in bioethics. Bioethics issues were cast not only in the context of the individual physician/patient encounter, but also in terms of encounters that did not typically raise immediate issues of serious physical risks to others. This myopia reached to the deepest theoretical levels, where basic normative commitments such as autonomy, and indeed the relationship between clinical medicine and public health, were understood simplistically, without appreciation of the moral significance of communicable infectious disease.

Public Health and Bioethics: Differing Paradigms

Ethical issues raised by infectious disease and transmissibility might seem properly to be the core domain of public health rather than part of the problems of clinical medicine that were the focus of bioethics. If so, it may seem unsurprising that bioethics ignored issues of infectiousness, perhaps working on the assumption that these issues were the province of a different field. Historically, infectious disease was indeed the staple issue of public health and continued to garner attention during the formative period of bioethics. But the discussions in public health at the time also were marked by optimism about infectious disease.

Long before the mechanisms of infectious disease transmission were understood, public health originated in societal attempts to try to control the spread of disease by isolating lepers, attaching bells to plague victims, imposing quarantines on ships entering a harbour (Venetian law reportedly required ships from the East to lie 40 days at anchor, hence the term 'quarantine'[8]), and similar measures. With increasing understanding of the microbial basis of infectious disease towards the end of the nineteenth century, practical public health measures became more effective, reflected in improved public sanitation, immunization, the application of the germ theory of disease in encouraging doctors to wash their hands between seeing patients, and many other public health measures aimed at reducing transmission. Indeed, at least until the mid-twentieth century, the containment of communicable infectious disease was the central concern of public health.

For the most part, public health has been population-focused rather than individual-focused, involving societal, governmental, or institutional measures aimed at protecting or improving the health of populations by containing or preventing transmission of disease rather than treating disease in individual patients. The generally accepted short definition of the field was formulated by the Institute of Medicine: 'what we, as a society, do collectively to assure the

[8] For a discussion of the history of quarantine, see the website of the US Centers for Disease Control, Division of Global Migration and Quarantine: http://www.cdc.gov/ncidod/dq/history.htm (accessed 24 February 2006).

conditions for people to be healthy'.[9] In a classic statement of the 'protean field of public health':

> Public Health is the science and art of preventing disease, prolonging life, and promoting physical health and efficiency through organized community effort for the sanitation of the environment, the control of communicable infections, the education of the individual in personal hygiene, the organization of medical and nursing services for the early diagnosis and preventive treatment of disease, and the development of the social machinery to insure everyone a standard of living adequate for the maintenance of health, so organizing these benefits as to enable every citizen to realize his birthright of health and longevity.[10]

Concomitantly, ethical paradigms in the field have been largely utilitarian in character, emphasizing protection of the community as a whole.[11] To be sure, public health has not ignored questions of distributive justice or even the treatment of disease in individual patients,[12] but its motivations for supporting health-improvement measures and for encouraging treatment have parallelled its motives for employing containment measures such as immunization and quarantine: to promote overall population health and to prevent the spread of the disease to other persons in the population as a whole. Public health is primarily concerned, in the common utilitarian view, with securing the greater overall good, even if that might involve unhappy tradeoffs for those comparatively few individuals who would be quarantined, forcibly immunized, isolated, or otherwise constrained.[13] To take just one example of the utilitarian theme in public health analyses, consider this quotation, from a widely-used public health text of the 1970s:

---

9 Institute of Medicine, *The Future of Public Health* (Washington, DC: National Academy Press, 1988): p. 19; also in the Preamble, *Principles of the Ethical Practice of Public Health* (American Society for Public Health, 2002) (http://www.apha.org/codeofethics/ethicsbrochure.pdf (accessed June 2006).

10 C.E.A. Winslow, 'The Untilled Fields of Public Health', *Science*, 51 (1920): 23, 30, quoted in W.K. Mariner, 'Law and Public Health: Beyond Emergency Preparedness', *Journal of Health Law*, 38 (2005): 251-2.

11 D.E. Beauchamp, 'Public Health: Alien Ethic in a Strange Land', *American Journal of Public Health*, 65 (1975): 1338-9.

12 Winslow, for example, wrote in 1920, that 'the public health worker needs the physician', and that 'such organized medical care must be made available not merely for the very poor and very right but for the entire community '. Winslow, 1920, p. 28.

13 See, e.g., D. Markovits, 'Quarantines and Distributive Justice', *Journal of Law, Medicine, & Ethics*, 33 (2005): 323-38; W.K. Mariner, 'Law and Public Health: Beyond Emergency Preparedness', *Journal of Health Law*, 38: (2005): 247-85; D. Callahan and B. Jennings, 'Ethics and Public Health: Forging a Strong Relationship', *American Journal of Public Health*, 92 (2002): 177-269.

> A large part of public health law in the United States is concerned with the control of communicable diseases. The most important basis on which rests the enactment and enforcement of public health law is the police power … It will suffice here to remind the reader of the folly, even in a democracy, of allowing individuals complete freedom of action. In fact individual freedom, in order truly to exist, must be limited to the right to engage in all activities except those that may be detrimental to the common welfare. An individual infected with a disease transmissible to others must necessarily forfeit some of his personal freedom for the common good.[14]

More recently, the *Principles of the Ethical Practice of Public Health* of the American Public Health Association contrasts the individual, provider-patient focus of clinical medicine with the population-based, prevention-emphasizing purview of public health.[15]

Bioethics, in contrast, was born at the bedside of the individual patient who is ill; it has been the illness of this patient and the way it affects him or her that has been the field's primary focus. Autonomy was the first of the four canonical principles in the field of bioethics, followed by nonmaleficence, beneficence, and justice; although this ordering was not meant to represent a prioritization, it nonetheless appears on the printed page almost uniformly in this order and has often been taken as a genuine priority-ranking in practice: autonomy has pride of place. Most forms of illness that concerned bioethics in its early days were not infectious, and, if infectious, were not addressed primarily with their potential for transmission in mind. The focus of bioethics has been the plight of *this* patient suffering *this* illness, and how this patient's interactions with physicians and others involved in decision-making about his or her care should go. To put the contrast in a nutshell, bioethics has been primarily interested in the patient as *victim*, public health in the patient as *vector*.

Perhaps contributing to this difference in focus, the field of bioethics developed in a manner that was for the most part institutionally independent of the field of public health. Bioethics grew up in schools of philosophy, theology, and in medical schools; schools of public health were institutionally distinct, often located at a distance, with comparatively little crossover in courses of study or faculty. Robert Veatch's history of the disrupted dialogue between humanists and physicians—as well as its reconnection in the 1970s—contains only a single mention of bioethics appointments in schools of public health—the appointment at the Harvard School of Public Health of two scholars associated with the Harvard Divinity School, Arthur Dyck and Ralph Potter—notably, to work on moral issues of policies related to fertility and migration.[16] A handful of well-known contemporary bioethicists

14 J.J. Hanlon, *Public Health Administration and Practice*, sixth edn (St. Louis: The C.V. Mosby Co., 1974): p. 401.

15 http://www.apha.org/codeofethics/ethicsbrochure.pdf (accessed June 2006).

16 R. Veatch, *Disrupted Dialogue: Medical Ethics and the Collapse of Physician-Humanist Communication* (New York, Oxford University Press 2005).

like Ruth Faden and Jeffrey Botkin and health lawyers such as George Annas and Wendy Mariner have degrees in public health, but this has not been the norm. Perhaps the most longstanding relationships between bioethics and public health ethics have been located at the Department of Health Law, Bioethics, and Human Rights at Boston University, founded in the 1980s,[17] and at Columbia University's Mailman School of Public Health, where Ronald Bayer is located. The entry of the Bloomberg School of Public Health at Johns Hopkins University is a relatively later development in the field, and the Phoebe R. Berman Bioethics Institute, affiliated with the School and now a leading supporter of work in bioethics, was not founded until 1995.[18] The migration of well-known bioethics scholars Dan Brock, Norman Daniels, and Dan Wikler to the Harvard School of Public Health is a twenty-first- century phenomenon.

The Shifting Concerns of Public Health

Public health measures have been astonishingly successful in transforming morbidity and mortality, especially for the developed world: up through the middle of the nineteenth century most people in most parts of the world died of infectious disease. By 1984, just before the outbreak of AIDS, infectious diseases—with the exception of pneumonia and septicemia—were no longer the leading causes of death in the developed world. They had been displaced by heart and circulatory disease, cancer, and various forms of degenerative organ system failure.

In more recent years, public health has increasingly turned its attention to other factors affecting the health of populations—matters like asbestos exposure, cigarette smoking, toxic waste, and obesity. While human behaviour plays a major role in these conditions, none of them involves biologically transmissible disease. Indeed, we can document for public health some of the same optimism that infectious disease had been conquered that we have already shown to pervade the development of the field of bioethics. During the formative period of bioethics—from the late 1950s to the advent of HIV/AIDS, attention in public health, too, was to some extent pointed away from infectious disease. This affected discussions in public health ethics, just as it did in bioethics.

This change in focus within public health is displayed, for example, in the classic public-health text, *Maxcy-Rosenau*, now in its fourteenth edition. The volume, reissued approximately every eight years, is a compendium of articles on topics in public health written by authorities in the field. The eighth edition, dating from 1956, devotes nearly six hundred pages to the prevention of communicable diseases, without discernable attention to ethical issues such as confidentiality

[17] The Department's website describes it as having been active for 'more than two decades'. http://www.bu.edu/dbin/sph/departments/health_law/research.php (accessed May 2006).

[18] See http://www.hopkinsmedicine.org/bioethics/about.html (accessed May 2006).

in the investigation and control of disease spread.[19] By 1978, the tenth edition, though featuring a new section on population dynamics, devoted fewer than five hundred pages to communicable diseases, again with no attention to the ethical issues they raise.[20]

The first entry in *Maxcy-Rosenau* specifically devoted to ethics and public health law appears in the eleventh edition, dated 1980. This entry is nothing short of remarkable. First, it attributes the importance of attending to a legal framework for public health activities to the movement in public health from disease prevention to health promotion and access to health services.[21] It treats the use of traditional methods of infection control such as quarantine and surveillance with breathtaking brevity. Ironically, this optimistic observation was published in 1980, scarcely a year before the initial reports of puzzling cases of immune-deficiency were published:

> Except for [tuberculosis and venereal diseases], measures to control reservoirs of infection tend not to be utilized. With most of the infectious diseases having been brought under control and with increased effectiveness of treatment resulting from the advent of antibiotics, the right to the individual to be free to move about at will took precedence over the needs to restrict him in the interest of protecting the public as a whole.[22]

Instead, the bulk of the discussion attends to the issues of paternalism and restrictions on liberty attendant on such public health interventions as cigarette smoking or exposure to toxic substances.

By the thirteenth edition of *Maxcy-Rosenau* in 1992, communicable diseases had shrunk to just over three hundred pages in the volume. Environmental health occupied almost four hundred pages; behavioural health, chronic illness and disability another almost four hundred. The final essay—a mere ten pages in the nearly 1200-page volume, is devoted to 'ethics and public health policy'. It reviews the canonical principles of bioethics—autonomy, beneficence, nonmaleficence, and justice—as helpful in public health dilemmas. The overall perspective of the analysis is that the rights of individuals must be balanced against the needs of communities, both where diseases are communicable and where they are not. More specifically, the author of this essay, John Last, suggests that 'a useful guideline is to consider the ethical principles of beneficent truth telling, distributive justice, and

---

19 K. Maxcy-Rosenau (ed.), *Maxcy-Rosenau Preventive Medicine and Public Health*, eighth edn (New York: Appleton Century Crofts, 1956).

20 P.E. Sartwell (ed.), *Maxcy-Rosenau Preventive Medicine and Public Health*, tenth edn (New York: Appleton Century Crofts, 1973).

21 Sidney Shindell, 'Legal and Ethical Aspects of Public Health', in J.A. Last & P.E. Sartwell (eds), *Maxcy-Rosenau Preventive Medicine and Public Health*, eleventh edn (New York: Appleton Century Crofts, 1980): pp. 1834-45.

22 Shindell, 1980, p. 1837.

nonmaleficence: what is the truth about the situation and which of the competing priorities will harm the fewest people over the longest period?'.[23]

This relative over-simplification of ethical issues in public health was not the full story. Appreciation of the tension between the contrasting paradigms of utilitarianism and respect for individuals appeared in the literature, both in discussions of behavioural interventions[24] and in discussions of research ethics.[25] Regular columns in the *American Journal of Public Health*, by William Curran, George Annas, Leonard Glantz, Ronald Bayer, and others, treated issues of law, ethics and public health, such as workplace hazards, abortion rights, and patient dumping. In the decades since the appearance of HIV/AIDS, these discussions have become far more robust.

At least three trends have become increasingly apparent in the more recent public health literature. One is the continuing debate about whether public health should confine itself to problems that are in some sense 'collective': problems of infection, sanitation, environmental hazards, and the like. Issues of population health—conditions that affect many in the population, such as obesity and diabetes, lack of exercise, and smoking—encompass far more than these collective problems, and have garnered as much attention in the public health literature as they have in the popular press. This approach has been picked up in bioethics as well, with scholars such as Dan Brock and Dan Wikler urging bioethics to take a 'bird's eye' view of ethics in healthcare.[26] The first of the anthologies to address ethics and public health directly, Dan Beauchamp and Bonnie Steinbock's *New Ethics for the Public's Health* (1999), devotes only four of its twenty-nine essays exclusively to infectious diseases, with human rights, access to healthcare, obesity, drug use, violent injury, gene therapy, infertility, tobacco, alcohol, and criminal justice occupying large sections of the volume.[27] Critics such as Richard

---

[23] J. Last, 'Ethics and Public Health Policy', in J.M. Last and R.B. Wallace (eds), *Maxcy-Rosenau-Last Public Health & Preventive Medicine*, thirteenth edn (Norwalk, CT: Appleton & Lange, 1992): pp. 1187-96.

[24] See, e.g., D.E. Beauchamp, 'Public Health: Alien Ethic in a Strange Land', *American Journal of Public Health*, 65 (1975): 1338-9.

[25] See, e.g., C.E. Lewis, M.A. Lewis and M. Ifekwunigue, 'Informed Consent by Children and Participation in an Influenza Vaccine Trial', *American Journal of Public Health*, 68/11 (1978): 1079-83; M.E. Martin, 'Statisticians, Confidentiality, and Privacy', *American Journal of Public Health*, 67/2 (1977): 165-7.

[26] D. Brock and D. Wikler, presentation at the International Association of Bioethics, Sydney, Australia, November 2004. Subsequently published as: D. Wikler & D. Brock, 'Population-Level Bioethics: Mapping a New Agenda' in A. Dawson, & M. Verweij (eds) *Ethics, Prevention, and Public Health* (Oxford: Oxford University Press, 2007).

[27] D.E. Beauchamp and B. Steinbock (eds), *New Ethics for the Public's Health* (Oxford: Oxford University Press, 1999).

Epstein have decried the implicit paternalism of public health efforts to improve population health through behaviour change.[28]

A second trend in public health is the move beyond 'international health', the effort to stop the spread of disease across national borders; to 'global health', the effort to address the overall burden of disease world-wide. Linkages between health and international human rights, drawn by Jonathan Mann,[29] Paul Farmer[30] and others in the fight against HIV/AIDS, drug-resistant tuberculosis, and the myriad diseases of poverty have greatly enriched recent ethics discussions in public health. The major impetus for this linkage between international human rights and global health has been renewed focus on the burdens of infectious disease in impoverished areas of the world,[31] including the efforts of Mann at UNAIDS and of Farmer in Haiti. Some theorists have gone so far as to argue that global disparities in health and human rights go hand in hand.[32] The journal *Health and Human Rights* (published since 1994), the creation of centres such as the François-Xavier Bagnoud Center for Health and Human Rights at Harvard in 1993 and the Center for Public Health and Human Rights at Johns Hopkins in 2004, and the devotion of a chapter in the *Oxford Textbook of Public Health*[33] to human rights all testify to the burgeoning role played by international human rights in the discipline of public health. In the United States, Larry Gostin has pressed the role of international human rights in protecting persons with HIV and the importance of civil rights in constructing a framework for domestic public health law.[34]

A third development in public health has been the field's self-conscious attention to its own ethical principles. Along with growth in public health education came attention to whether schools of public health taught ethics; in 1976, at least, the

---

[28] R.A. Epstein, 'In Defense of the "Old" Public Health: The Legal Framework for the Regulation of Public Health', *Brooklyn Law Review*, 69 (2004): 1421-70.

[29] J.M. Mann, 'Medicine and Public Health, Ethics and Human Rights', *Hastings Center Report* (1997): 6-13.

[30] P. Farmer, *Pathologies of Power: Health, Human Rights, and the New War on the Poor* (Berkeley, CA: University of California Press, 2005).

[31] T.M. Brown, M. Cueto, and E. Fee, 'The World Health Organization and the Transition from "International" to "Global" Public Health', *American Journal of Public Health*, 96 (2006): 62-72.

[32] S.R. Benatar, 'Global Disparities in Health and Human Rights: a Critical Commentary', *American Journal of Public Health*, 88/2 (1998): 295-300; M. Roemer and R. Roemer, 'Global health, national development, and the role of government', *American Journal of Public Health*, 80/10 (1990): 88-92.

[33] S. Gruskin and D. Tarantola, 'Health and Human Rights', Chapter. 4.1 in R. Detels, J. McEwen, R. Beaglehole and H. Tanada (eds), *Oxford Textbook of Public Health*, fourth edn (Oxford: Oxford University Press, 2002).

[34] L.O. Gostin and Z. Lazzarini, *Human Rights and Public Health in the AIDS Pandemic* (New York: Oxford University Press, 1997); L.O. Gostin, *Public Health Law: Power, Duty, Restraint* (Berkeley, CA: University of California Press, 2000).

answer was largely 'no',[35] but by 1999 all but two of 24 schools responding offered courses in the field.[36] In 2002, the American Public Health Association adopted a code of ethics, the *Principles of the Ethical Practice of Public Health*.[37] A primary rationale for this code of ethics was that the field of public health had treated ethical principles as implicit but needed to make them explicit and public. The code begins with the affirmation that human beings have a right to the resources necessary for health; it continues by asserting that humans are inherently interdependent and social values of trust, community, and participation are core ethical concerns. Development of the code was the occasion for systematic reflection on the ethical structure of public health[38] as well as calls for increased cooperation between the fields of public health ethics and bioethics.[39]

To sum up, until quite recently, public health ethics has not only been institutionally separate but has occupied a separate sphere of discussion from bioethics. This separateness may be a function of deeper incompatibilities between the conceptual and theoretical paradigms in use in the fields. Clinical ethics—the original core of bioethics—has been primarily based in a Kantian-influenced respect-for-persons view, in which principles like autonomy, truth-telling, confidentiality, informed consent, and other individual-centred, individual-respecting principles are central, while public health is rooted in a far more utilitarian, population-based, 'good-of-the-whole' ethical view.[40]

Closing the Gap: Convergence Between the Ethics of Public Health and Bioethics

In very recent years, the gap between bioethics and public health ethics has been closing. To some extent, this convergence has been stimulated by the self-conscious

35 N.R. Bluestone, 'The Teaching of Ethics in Schools of Public Health', *American Journal of Public Health*, 66/5 (1976): 478-9 (10-15 schools responding had no ethics course; only Harvard and Columbia indicated significant ethics offerings).

36 S.S. Coughlin, W.H. Katz, and D.R. Mattison, 'Ethics Instruction at Schools of Public Health in the United States', *American Journal of Public Health*, 89/5 (1999): 768-70.

37 http://www.apha.org/codeofethics/ethicsbrochure.pdf (accessed June 2006).

38 N.E. Kass, 'An Ethics Framework for Public Health', *American Journal of Public Health*, 91/11 (2001): 1776-82.

39 B. Wolder Levin and A.R. Fleishman, 'Public Health and Bioethics: The Benefits of Collaboration', *American Journal of Public Health*, 92 (2002): 165-7; D. Callahan and B. Jennings, 'Ethics and Public Health: Forging a Strong Relationship', *American Journal of Public Health* 92 (2002): 169-77.

40 This is the picture presented by Kass (2001).

attention to ethics by scholars in public health.[41] Work in bioethics, too, has begun to address points of contact between the fields, both in terms of particular issues and possibilities for theoretical convergence. There has been significant interest among the bioethics journals, as exhibited for example in the special issues of the *Journal of Law, Medicine and Ethics* (winter 2003 and its winter 2003 special supplement) devoted to population health and to public health and law, the issue of *Bioethics* devoted to public health in 2004,[42] and the issue of *Bioethics* devoted to infectious disease in 2005.[43]

These are but beginnings, however. To date, no fully systematic account has attempted to see whether the insights of one field warrant extensive reassessment of the other, in either direction. Instead, the picture remains one of the need to mediate the tensions between the individualism of bioethics and its privileging of autonomy on the one hand and the concern of public health for the good of all on the other. Ron Bayer and Amy Fairchild put it bluntly: 'As we commence the process of shaping an ethics of public health, it is clear that bioethics is the wrong place to start when thinking about the balances required in defense of the public's health'. This apparent gap between bioethics and public health, we believe, is exacerbated and reflected in the somewhat different ethical paradigms these fields employ, and it is part of our project to see whether the gap can be closed.

HIV 'Exceptionalism'

The link between bioethics and public health ethics first began to be forged when HIV/AIDS was emerging in the early 1980s. HIV was in some respects a wakeup call for bioethics, bringing a reinvigoration of traditional public health concerns about communicable disease.[44] In other respects, however, HIV may have been doubly 'exceptional', to use Ron Bayer's term, and thus not have been seen to pose the more thoroughgoing theoretical challenges to bioethics (and perhaps also to public health)

---

[41] Examples include D.E. Beauchamp and B. Steinbock (eds), *New Ethics for the Public's Health* (New York: Oxford University Press, 1999); S.S Coughlin, C. Soskolne, and K. Goodman (eds), *Case Studies in Public Health Ethics* (American Public Health Association, 1998); L.O. Gostin (ed.), *Public Health Law and Ethics* (Berkeley, CA: University of California Press, 2002); M. Boylan (ed.), *Public Health Policy and Ethics* (Dordrecht: Kluwer Academic Publishers, 2004); and A. Dawson & M. Verweij (eds), *Ethics, Prevention, and Public Health* (Oxford: Oxford University Press, 2007).

[42] W. Rogers and D. Brock (eds), 'Ethics and Public Health', special issue of *Bioethics*, 18/6 (November 2004).

[43] M.J. Selgelid and M.P. Battin (eds), 'Ethics and Infectious Disease' special issue of *Bioethics*, 19/4 (August 2005); also expanded as M.J. Selgelid, M.P. Battin, and C.B. Smith (eds), *Ethics and Infectious Disease* (Oxford: Blackwell, 2006).

[44] An excellent discussion of the ethical issues raised by HIV is R. Bayer, *Private Acts, Social Consequences* (New York: The Free Press, 1989).

that we explore in this volume. This is for several reasons, both biological and political. For one thing, the transmission routes of HIV infection—through the exchange of bodily fluids—are likely to be the subjects of both awareness and control. For another, the politics of HIV have been shaped by analyses framed in rights-based terms. In neither of these ways is HIV representative of the fuller range of infectious diseases.

HIV is transmissible only by routes that today can be largely brought under the control of the agent or identified others such as healthcare providers: primarily sexual intercourse, sharing of syringes in intravenous drug administration, and exposure to contaminated blood products or other bodily fluids such as semen. While HIV is like many other infectious diseases in that it can be (and very often is) transmitted unknowingly or unintentionally, the mechanisms of transmission are nevertheless open in principle to the agent's control, both for the transmitter and the transmittee, especially with adequate education. There are even reported incidents of quite deliberately conducted transmission of HIV, including a website for 'bugchasers' who wish to receive or transmit HIV.[45] This is quite a different picture from diseases that are aerosolized or transmitted through intermediate vectors like mosquitoes; here, the human agents—both transmitter and transmittee, even with the conscientious use of such measures as masks or bed nets—have very much less control over whether the disease is passed along. HIV is also quite different from diseases that have common reservoirs—water or soil—because these reservoirs are far less easy for ordinary people to avoid. Both vector-limitation and victim-protection are thus more easily constructed for HIV than for infectious diseases such as influenza. Moreover, these mechanisms of HIV transmission and prevention became known quite soon—within a few years—after the identification of the syndrome itself.

To say that HIV is in many ways exceptional is certainly not to say that there is a sharp distinction between HIV and other infectious diseases—they share many features—nor that HIV is fully unique. But the fact that the HIV virus is not transmitted casually or by diffuse routes such as aerosolization or intermediate vectors, but only by the limited routes of exchanges of bodily fluids normally subject to agent control is a very significant difference. Thus it may be especially telling that the first extensive efforts of modern bioethics to deal with an infectious disease were focused on HIV, one of the least instructive and least challenging cases for understanding the *theoretical* implications of infectious disease for bioethics more generally, despite its enormous and devastating global impact.

That HIV is transmitted by well-identified and potentially manageable routes has been an attractive draw for public health interventions in at least some countries. Cuba, for example, quarantined HIV+ persons and has comparatively

---

45 See 'Bugchasers: The men who long to be HIV+', *Rolling Stone* online, available at www.solargeneral.com/pdf/BugChasers.pdf (accessed 8 February 2006).

successfully contained the spread of the infection in that country.[46] Brazil has also been successful in controlling its epidemic, but using largely education rather than forcible constraint. There is much that could be said about the justice or injustice of various disease-control measures and constraints, but it is this feature of HIV that makes it seem more tractable to relatively straightforward public health interventions—testing, reporting, and restraining—than many other infectious diseases. Of course, claims that changing transmission behaviour is easier in HIV than for other infectious diseases may be culturally relative, but it is at a minimum true, that HIV is not contracted—as some infectious diseases are, like flu—just by walking around.

The pressures on confidentiality and on liberty presented by the possibility of effective public health interventions against HIV resulted in demands for the protection of civil liberties in countries such as the United States with strongly rights-protective regimes. These demands for rights-protections were greatly intensified by the overall climate of concern for civil rights generally and rights for sexual liberty more particularly that obtained during the late 1970s and early 1980s, the initial era of HIV.[47] Zita Lazzarini gives this account of the exceptionalism argument about HIV:

> Supposedly, the argument goes, public fear was so great, the political power of gay men so substantial, and concern over stigmatization and discrimination so real, that public health authorities abandoned "traditional" and effective approaches to communicable disease control in favour of a civil liberties-focused approach. This resulted in policies that emphasized pre- and post-test counseling, anonymous testing, and stringent protections of confidentiality as opposed to named reporting, targeted screening, and partner notification.[48]

Abigail Zuger identifies AIDS as the 'first disease on record to spawn a huge, vocal, visible, angry grass-roots patients' rights movement that changed the course of history'.[49] AIDS activists have been very effective in forcing public health officials and legislators to consider the rights of patients to privacy, autonomous decision making regarding their care, and the rights of infected patients to justice in the distribution of healthcare resources. Conversely, the relation of AIDS communicability to specific human behaviours has forced individual practitioners

46 For a sympathetic account of Cuban HIV policy, see P. Farmer, *Pathologies of Power: Health, Human Rights, and the New War on the Poor* (Berkeley, CA: University of California Press, 2005), especially, Chapter 2.

47 The United States Centers for Disease Control (CDC) identified the syndrome in 1981; the virus was identified in 1984.

48 Z. Lazzarini, 'What Lessons Can We Learn from the Exceptionalism Debate (Finally)?', *Journal of Law, Medicine & Ethics*, 29 (2001): 149-51.

49 A. Zuger, 'What did we learn from AIDS?', *New York Times* (11 November 2003): p.D6.

to be more open about questioning patients' private behaviours, to be more concerned with educating patients and the public about high risk behaviours and to consider classical public health methods for reducing communicability. In many ways, AIDS and many other infectious diseases require us to consider the patient as both a *victim* with individual needs and rights and as a potential *vector* of disease that is of concern to the community.[50] But the way in which a person contracting AIDS is a victim and that same person transmitting AIDS is a vector is different from many other forms of communicable infectious disease.

At the time HIV came on the scene, there was increased legal emphasis on liberty in intimate sexual relationships. The initial primary mode of transmission that introduced HIV into the United States—sexual activity among gay men—made it seem particularly difficult to regulate. Ron Bayer pointed out quite early in the discussions of HIV that it was being treated differently from other infectious diseases, with an emphasis on individual rights, for example on counselling before testing. Bayer describes in extensive and regretful detail how gay activism made it difficult even to regulate the bath houses in San Francisco and New York that were a major locus of HIV transmission.[51] Bayer is very sensitive to the ironies of the interventions that would be required for survival, just when gay men were achieving freedom, as well as to the disastrous risks of stigmatization given ongoing attitudes about gay sexuality. At the same time, Bayer relates, the public health law of disease control was mired in the turn of the preceding century, in yellow fever and quarantine cases where state power had been left relatively unfettered regardless of the rationale for the intervention. Even with modern due process law, however, Bayer believes that there are important conflicts between civil rights (including individual choices about intimate behaviour) and the fact that efforts to stop the spread of this deadly disease would have required decisions to change intimate behaviour. A full account of ethics in infectious disease must explore whether this conflictual view—sexual liberty over against the protection of the community—is too limited; we believe that it is.

More recently, as HIV has come to be thought of as a chronic disease in areas of the world where effective anti-retroviral therapy is available; there have been calls for its 'normalization'.[52] Examples of such normalization include routine reporting, contact tracing, routine prenatal testing, home over-the-counter test kits, and the use of rapid tests not requiring long waiting periods for results. There have, however, been calls for the reintroduction of the fully utilitarian paradigms

---

50 J.M. Mann, 'Medicine and Public Health, Ethics and Human Rights', *The Hastings Center Reports*, 27(3) (1997): 6-13.

51 Bayer, especially Chapter 2.

52 See, e.g., R. Bayer, 'Public Health Policy and the AIDS Epidemic: An End to HIV Exceptionalism?', *New England Journal of Medicine*, 324 (1991): 1500-504; Bayer, 'Clinical Progress and the Future of HIV Exceptionalism', *Archives of Internal Medicine*, 159 (1999): 1042-8; L.F. Ross, 'Genetic Exceptionalism vs. Paradigm Shift: Lessons from HIV', *Journal of Law, Medicine & Ethics*, 29 (2001): 141-6.

of public health, such as mandatory testing and contact-tracing, as HIV rates have begun to increase.[53]

To be sure, bioethics developed tremendously in response to the crisis of HIV/AIDS. Discussions of issues like obligations to treat, personal responsibility for disease, confidentiality, public surveillance, justice in international research, and the stigmatization of gay men and intravenous drug users have assumed great importance in bioethics. The growth in bioethics has been extraordinary; but these concerns have still been largely discussed within the traditional framework of bioethics, based in liberal theory and its standard constructions of autonomy and the harm principle. What these discussions have not taken fully into account has been characterized as the dual exceptionalism of AIDS: its mode of transmission and the rights-activism which accompanied it. HIV/AIDS has not presented the full range of challenges other infectious diseases might to standard liberal paradigms in bioethics. Thus the conclusions reached in bioethics about HIV/AIDS have not been—and could not easily have been—extended to infectious disease as a whole, as we documented earlier in this chapter. Recent calls for the normalization of responses to HIV and for the application of public health ethics to the case of HIV may prove useful, but are, we think, also incomplete. They, too, require development of the more robust structures for bioethical analysis.

Looking Ahead

In understanding the ethical implications of communicable infectious disease, we believe, something is needed in between the familiar postures of bioethics and of public health. The patient is a current victim of infectious disease; the patient is also a potential vector of infectious disease, but in order to be able to see this person in both ways at once, we believe, we require a revised theoretical paradigm, one that can make possible a genuine union or at least a real connection possible between the sort of traditional clinical medicine that has been the concern of bioethics and the population-wide view that has been the concern of public health. A revised theoretical paradigm, as we are in the process of developing, must be capable of seeing the patient in *both ways at once*—not just flipping back and forth from one view to the other. Both public health ethics and bioethics will gain, we believe, not so much by replacing the basic paradigm of bioethics with that of public health, or the other way around, but by modifying and enhancing what each has developed so far. Both fields require rethinking of basic theoretical notions—autonomy, the individual patient, the harm principle, the public—in light of the idea that we are all, always, in some sense victims and vectors to each other. To be sure, some

53 See, e.g., J.F. Dobkin, 'HIV Management: Time for a Public Health Approach?', *Infections in Medicine*, 23 (2006): 48-9; T.R. Frieden, M. Das-Douglas, S.E. Kellerman, and K.J. Henning, 'Applying Public Health Principles to the HIV Epidemic', *New England Journal of Medicine*, 353/22 (2005): 2397-402.

attempted fusions of moral concerns are best described, as Mark Sagoff puts it, as 'bad marriage, quick divorce',[54] but other deep-level fusions are fruitful indeed, and we think that this is possible—indeed, urgent—between bioethics and public health.

[54] Sagoff's reference is to environmental ethics and animal rights. See M. Sagoff, 'Animal Liberation and Environmental Ethics: Bad Marriage, Quick Divorce', *Osgoode Hall, LJ*, 22 (1984): 297.

Chapter 15
The Common Good Argument and HIV Prevention

Charlotte Paul
Otago University, New Zealand

On the face of it, it is puzzling that despite the clear relationship between increasing numbers of sexual partners and HIV risk, framing prevention advice in terms of partner reduction remains highly contested. When epidemiologists in the United States first described the sexual behaviours fuelling the epidemic there were accusations of closet moralism; understandable in the climate of the time when gay men feared being 'pathologized' again.[1] But more recently, an explicit focus on reducing number of sexual partners (among other matters) to control the HIV epidemic in countries in Africa has been widely criticized. Medical anthropologist Edward Green has responded, 'Where is the risk of warning about the dangers of having multiple partners in a pandemic driven by having multiple partners?'.[2]

The effect of reducing numbers of sexual partners can be conceived both as a way of protecting the individual and of protecting the group. The latter I have called the common good argument; that is the argument that people have an interest held in common in protecting their community from HIV. In what follows I outline why protection of the group is important, describe ideas about the common good, and illustrate their implications for the methods and ethics of HIV prevention. I explore the reasons why this common good approach is still beset with problems and finally propose a way in which it might be taken forward. The paper draws on epidemiological information that will be familiar to those working in the field. I have drawn on one source in particular for the idea of a sexual ecology and what it might mean.[3]

---

1 R. Bayer, *Private Acts, Social Consequences: AIDS and the Politics of Public Health* (New York: The Free Press, 1989), p. 26.

2 E.C. Green, *Rethinking AIDS Prevention* (Westport, CT: Praeger, 2003).

3 G. Rotello, *Sexual Ecology: AIDS and the Destiny of Gay Men* (New York: Plume, 1998).

Why an Interest Held in Common in HIV Prevention Makes Epidemiological Sense

The risk of acquiring HIV depends on whether one's partner has HIV, which in turn depends on the prevalence of HIV in the relevant community. This can be illustrated from data on acquisition of herpes simplex type 2 (HSV-2), another sexually acquired chronic viral infection, in a birth cohort—at ages 21, 26 and 32 years. Prevalence rises with age in the cohort—for women from less than 5 per cent at age 21 to 23 per cent at age 32. The risk per sexual partnership of acquiring HSV-2 is two and three times as high from 26 to 32 years as from first coitus up to age 26—for women and men respectively.[4]

It is similar, over time, for HIV epidemics. There is less risk of acquiring HIV through an 'unsafe' sexual partnership early in an epidemic than later, i.e. when prevalence is low vs. high. Hence there is a community interest in HIV prevention. To put it another way: prevalence drives incidence; if prevalence is low, there is less chance of any individual becoming infected.

Secondly, epidemic spread at the beginning depends on the basic reproductive rate (or number), *Ro*, which is the average number of new infections produced when one infected individual is introduced into a population. This in turn depends on three parameters: the transmission probability per partner, the number of new sexual partners per unit time, and the average duration of the infectious period.[5] Modelling approaches have shown that small changes in the average number of sexual partners can push *Ro* over 1, such that epidemic spread occurs, and this can lead to a major change in prevalence. For instance, in the mid-1990s, a model based on data from gay men in New York showed that one additional 'unsafe' partnership per year on average would push transmission above the threshold and lead to a major increase in incidence and prevalence. This has been described as an example of the 'tragedy of the commons.'[6] The increment in individual risk from a slight increase in contact rate is negligible, assuming the individual acts alone. But if all individuals make this choice, the aggregate impact is a phase shift in the population dynamics of the disease, dramatically increasing everyone's risk. The metaphor was first used in an ecological sense in relation to environmental degradation and over-population in the 1960s.[7] Avoiding tragedy depends on shared restraint, not on individual choice.

---

4 N. Dickson, T. Van Roode, P. Herbison, et al., 'Risk of HSV-2 acquisition increases over early adulthood: evidence from a cohort study', *Sexually Transmitted Infections*, 83 (2007): 87-90.

5 R.M. Anderson and R.M. May, *Infectious Diseases of Humans: Dynamics and Control* (New York: Oxford University Press, 1991).

6 Rotello, *Sexual Ecology*; M. Morris and L. Dean, 'Effect of sexual behaviour change on long-term Human Immunodeficiency Virus Prevalence among homosexual men', *American Journal of Epidemiology*, 140 (1994): 217-32.

7 G. Hardin, 'The tragedy of the commons', *Science*, 162 (1968): 1243-8.

Thirdly, it is a truism in public health that the population level of a behaviour affects the proportion of people who are at the extreme end of the distribution. (This is true even when the high values are removed when calculating averages.) For instance in the case of alcohol, there is evidence that a drinker's risk of becoming a heavy drinker depends on the 'wetness' of the drinking culture to which the individual belongs.[8] Similarly the prevalence of obesity is a function of the population's average weight. Rose has suggested that the problems of any minority—drug users or criminals or the homeless or the mentally ill—should be understood in reference to the whole society. When social risk factors change, their distribution tends to shift as a whole, reflecting the coherent nature of society.[9] For sexual behaviour, this has been little explored. Nevertheless there is evidence that the major changes in sexual behaviour that have accompanied changes in sexual mores over the last 40 years in Western countries have been evident not only in an increased proportion reporting large numbers of sexual partners but also in major changes in the proportions reporting one or two partners.[10]

What is the Common Good?

Beauchamp has described the common good in public health as referring to the welfare of individuals considered as a group: the body politic. His view draws on traditions which see the good of society as more than the sum of individual goods, and where that good is expressed through practices.[11] It is the idea that the public is presumed to have an interest, held in common, in prevention of threats to their welfare. The bioethicist, Callahan, describes attention to the common good as a way of framing issues or questions: for instance, 'what will x mean for all of us together?'[12] To frame a question in this way is (a) to take an ethical position: that the common good matters, not just individual good and that solidarity—acting together to achieve common goals—matters; and (b) to recognize an empirical fact about public health. This fact is most obvious in matters that lead to social disruption. It is less obvious, but as I have shown, just as true, for HIV prevention.

---

8 G. Rose, *The Strategy of Preventive Medicine* (Oxford: Oxford University Press, 1992).

9 Rose, *The Strategy of Preventive Medicine.*

10 C. Paul, N. Dickson, P.B. Davis, et al., 'Heterosexual behaviour and HIV risk in New Zealand: data from a national survey', *Australian Journal of Public Health*, 19 (1995): 13-18.

11 D. Beauchamp, 'Community: The neglected tradition of public health', in L.O. Gostin (ed.) *Public Health Law and Ethics: a Reader* (Berkeley, CA: University of California Press, 2002).

12 D. Callahan, 'Individual good and common good: a communitarian approach to bioethics', *Perspectives in Biology and Medicine*, 46 (2003): 496-507.

Implications for HIV Prevention

To be most effective, HIV prevention measures should recognize the way in which everyone's behaviour matters. In this it is similar to other public health issues such as immunization. For some diseases, when immunization coverage is high, the disease will die out but when coverage is only moderate, the age of attack will be raised. For example for rubella, a girl not immunized will grow up quite safe when immunization coverage is high. But the same child, if immunization coverage is moderate, will be at *greater* risk of growing up to suffer a rubella infection in pregnancy (i.e. to contract the disease at an older age) than if no one in the community had been immunized at all.[13] Prevention calls for collective responsibility. Rose quotes Dostoevsky: 'We are all responsible for all'.[14]

At the least, each individual has an interest in other individuals (and not just their own partner) behaving safely—for instance using condoms. This also means that all individuals should have an interest in changing group norms towards safety. This is fairly uncontroversial. For instance, in New Zealand the AIDS Foundation has worked hard over many years to promote a condom culture among gay men.

But in the long term more than a condom strategy is required. With new 'technological' ways of reducing risk of HIV transmission—e.g. condoms, treatment of HIV with antiretrovirals—have come compensatory increases in unsafe sexual behaviour, sparked by decreases in perceived risk. This has been called 'risk compensation'.[15]

It is plausible that more fundamental changes in the culture in which such risk behaviour takes place could shift population norms towards safety in relation to other aspects of sexual behaviour; in particular the number of sexual partners.

The gay journalist Gabriel Rotello, writing about gay men in the US, uses the environmentalists' language of 'sustainablity'.[16] He asserts that every society on record has attempted to channel sexual desire in ways that promote stability. For him, imagining a sustainable sexual culture for gay men entails providing the conditions in which self-imposed sexual restraint might become the norm. In a similar way, new public health models of the determinants of HIV risk emphasize cultural and political context alongside social and structural factors such as discrimination and the disruption caused by war.[17]

---

13 T. Panagiotopoulos, I. Antoniadou and E. Valassi-Adam, 'Increase in congenital rubella occurrence after immunization in Greece: retrospective survey and systematic review', *British Medical Journal*, 319 (1999): 1462-7.

14 Rose, *The Strategy of Preventive Medicine*.

15 M.M. Cassell, D.T. Halperin, J.D. Shelton and D. Stanton, 'Risk compensation: the Achilles' heel of innovations in HIV prevention', *British Medical Journal*, 332 (2006): 605-7.

16 Rotello, *Sexual Ecology*.

17 K.E. Poundstone, S.A. Strathdee and D.D. Celentano, 'The social epidemiology of Human Immunodeficiency Virus/Acquired Immunodeficiency Syndrome', *Epidemiologic Reviews*, 26 (2004): 22-35.

In relation to generalized heterosexual epidemics in a number of countries, where there have been successes in reducing HIV transmission, a major contribution appears to have been made by a reduction in the number of sexual partnerships. The decline in HIV prevalence (and incidence) in Uganda has focused international attention on what has been called 'Primary Behaviour Change': delay in first sex and reduction in number of sexual partnerships.[18] [19] [20] The rhetoric has been explicitly about the common good. A widely used metaphor was the hungry lion that had entered the village; people must act together to protect the village and the nation.[21] As Michael Cassell and colleagues said:

> The experience of Uganda suggests that by working with individuals, leaders, and institutions throughout communities, we can help foster and reinforce shared perceptions that certain risk behaviours are both personally unwise and raise the burden and effects of disease for all.[22]

New empirical evidence for the continuing role of multiple partners among homosexual men in the US comes from a study of 3,000 men which showed that a major independent risk factor for HIV transmission was greater numbers of sexual partners.[23] Finally, it makes public health sense to have *more* than one strategy. Nevertheless, while most experts accept that partner reduction makes epidemiological sense, it has been claimed that 'partner reduction is good epidemiology not good ideology'.[24]

Implications for the Ethics of Prevention

It is clear that the realities of HIV transmission and the desire to prevent it inevitably link individual sexual behaviour with the good of the whole. This should mean that partner reduction is good ideology (or ethics) as well as good

---

18 Green, *Rethinking AIDS Prevention.*

19 E.C. Green, D.T. Halperin, V. Nantulya and J.A. Hogle, 'Uganda's HIV prevention success: the role of sexual behaviour change and the national response', *AIDS and Behaviour*, 10/4 (2006): 335-46.

20 J.D. Shelton, D.T. Halperin, V. Nantulya, et al., 'Partner reduction is crucial for balanced "ABC" approach to HIV prevention', *British Medical Journal*, 328 (2004): 848-9.

21 Green, *Rethinking AIDS Prevention.*

22 Cassell et al., 'Risk compensation'.

23 S.P. Buchbinder, E. Vittinghoff, P.J. Heagerty, et al., 'Sexual risk, nitrite inhalant use, and lack of circumcision associated with HIV seroconversion in men who have sex with men in the United States', *Journal of Acquired Immune Deficiency Syndrome*, 39 (2005): 82-9.

24 D. Wilson, 'Partner reduction and the prevention of HIV/AIDS', *British Medical Journal*, 328 (2004): 848-9.

epidemiology. Rotello has described the way in which the morality of an act can be seen to depend on the state of the system at the time.[25] Harm is the key. When a high average number of sexual partners tips the balance to raise the prevalence of disease among the 'commons' then there is a moral obligation towards sexual restraint. Sustaining a culture of restraint entails changing the environment to support long-term relationships as well as to support condom use. Similarly in a heterosexual epidemic, 'primary' changes in sexual behaviour such as delaying first sex and reducing number of partners (as well as condom use) might then be subject to a moral obligation.

Problems with the Common Good Approach

There are a number of important criticisms of HIV prevention approaches based on advocacy of cultural change towards restraint.

Firstly, the use of words that convey a moral obligation within intimate relationships can carry an explosive charge and lead to accusations of moralism, especially among those whose sexual behaviour has been stigmatized. For instance, Rottello was unambiguous that his morality *didn't* imply that 'monogamy' was better than 'promiscuity' in general. It was only so in the context of an HIV epidemic; the moral imperative was simply to prevent spread. Even so he was accused of having a hidden agenda of moralism and even of homophobia.[26]

In a similar way the ABC approach (Abstinence, Be faithful, use Condoms) first used in Botswana[27] has been widely criticized, as has the similar primary behaviour change approach used in Uganda. A spokeswoman for the UK charity Christian Aid has described good reasons why they had rejected ABC in favour of SAVE (Safer practices, Available medications, Voluntary counselling and testing, Empowerment). In Christian Aid's view ABC can add to stigma. But she concluded: 'HIV is a virus, not a moral issue. The response to HIV must be based on public health measures and human rights principles'.[28]

The common good argument requires that people make moral decisions about sex on the basis of protecting each other and the community from infection. But there are, of course, other moral dimensions to sexual behaviour and critics may worry that to discuss a moral dimension at all is to confuse private and public issues. For instance moral views on exploitation and objectification and on love have not much to do with sexual transmission of infection nor, necessarily, with

---

[25] Rotello, *Sexual Ecology*.

[26] Ibid.

[27] AVERT, 'The ABC of HIV prevention': http://www.avert.org/abc-hiv.htm (accessed 20 October 2007).

[28] R. Baggaley, 'SAVE: Christian Aid's new strategy to fight AIDS', *The Pop Reporter* 18 March 2006 (15 June 2006), http://www.infoforhealth.org/popreporter (accessed May 2006).

number of partners or age at first sex. Then there is the rule-based morality of certain religious traditions. The vehicle for the common good ideas in Uganda has been the religious language of chastity and faithfulness.

The Christian Aid spokesperson said that HIV is not a moral issue (though she uses the moral language of human rights). I assume she says HIV is not a moral issue because to her 'moral' means this rule-based morality. Alternatively she may believe that telling people how to behave in intimate relationships is itself seen as morally wrong—according to a human rights perspective. Whichever reason applies, by using traditional moral language, the ABC approach seems to blur distinctions among moral sources. Yet the two moral sources of the common good and the religious rule are not so far apart. Moral proscriptions around sex must have their origins partly in concerns about disease. Moreover, faithfulness is just a promise and has no necessary religious roots.

Secondly, it has been widely regarded as unworkable in practice, despite the evidence. On this view, only technological solutions such as condoms or circumcision or vaccines that do not require fundamental changes in behaviour can realistically alter the spread of HIV. This is the conventional liberal position. Strongly polarized views, particularly in the US, about young people and sex education: the so called 'culture wars' which pit abstinence against condoms, have made it difficult to consider the evidence impartially. If anyone supports a role for abstinence they may be accused of joining the religious conservatives. On the other side, the US government has required recipients of grants for HIV prevention to sign a 'loyalty oath' opposing prostitution—making it in effect impossible to educate sex workers on HIV transmission.[29]

It is important to note that effective changes incorporating this common good approach entailed more than exhortations to care for each other and the community. It has also entailed modifications to the culture and environment to support primary behaviour change. For instance in Uganda:

> Linked to high-level political support and grassroots-level communications for behaviour change was a strong emphasis on greater empowerment of women and girls; targeting youth both in and out of school; and aggressively fighting stigma and discrimination against people living with HIV/AIDS.[30]

It has been argued that these combined initiatives have led to such radical changes in sexual behaviour that they amount to a 'social vaccine'—of similar impact to a vaccine of 80 per cent efficacy.[31]

---

[29] Comment and Analysis, 'HIV/AIDS: We must simply tell it like it is', *Guardian Weekly* (June 9-15 2006): 13.

[30] Shelton et al., 'Partner reduction is crucial'.

[31] R.L. Stoneburner and D. Low-Beer, 'Population-level HIV declines and behavioural risk avoidance in Uganda', *Science*, 304 (2004): 714-18.

Thirdly, the common good argument is not just about self-protection but also about protection of the other. Hence it entails obligations on people who are infected and this has been characterized as blaming the victim. If infected people are already marginalized or stigmatized, such obligations can seem, not as if the society is sharing their burden, but as if they are being given a disproportionate burden. Moreover, in its emphasis on faithfulness, it fails to consider the power imbalances within heterosexual relationships. Where women have little power, and when the greatest risk for HIV is getting married, calls for faithfulness may not help.

Even this objection does not seem to be insurmountable. In fact the victim is more to blame in an individual rights model. In a common good model, the responsibilities are on everyone, infected and not infected, to consider others. Ways to address stigma and discrimination must go along with education as they apparently have in Uganda. Condom promotion (or in the future microbicides) must go along with A and B (of the ABC approach) as must empowerment of women and legal protections against coerced sex. Moreover, the problems, such as lack of equality for women, which could hinder the success of measures to delay first sex or reduce numbers of partners, are also likely to hinder the use of condoms.[32] Legal protections and incentives for gay men to have the same opportunities for social/sexual stability as heterosexuals (e.g. gay marriage) are built into the idea of a sustainable gay sexual ecology.[33]

Fourthly, there is the question, whose commons? Is it wrong for an outsider to presume to write about gay men in the US or about people in countries affected by generalized heterosexual epidemics? I am of course quoting people in those communities and close observers of them. But should anyone outside the 'commons' speak? Is even quoting the voices of others a problem? It may even be argued that sexual minorities don't share the same commons with the privileged majority. I think this requires great sensitivity but should not be seen as a complete obstacle. Ultimately we are all part of the same commons.

The final problem is of competing and possibly incompatible conceptions of the moral life. The common good isn't part of the dominant moral language in many industrialized countries. The 'first language' of political individualism and rights[34] [35] is so dominant. The 'second language' of the common good is hard to articulate. Moreover, individualism pursued as a dominant value has weakened the force of calls for collective responsibility. The unfettered pursuit of individualism

32 J. De Irala and A. Alonso, 'Changes in sexual behaviours to prevent HIV', *Lancet*, 368 (2006): 1749-50.

33 Rotello, *Rethinking AIDS Prevention*.

34 R. Bellah, R. Madsen, W. Sullivan, A. Swidler and S. Tipton, *Habits of the Heart: Individualism and Commitment in American Life* (Berkley, CA: University of California Press, 1985).

35 L. Wallack and R. Lawrence, 'Talking about public health: developing America's "Second Language"', *American Journal of Public Health*, 45 (2005): 567-70.

over the last 30 years and the growth in inequality which has accompanied it may also have weakened the coherent nature of the societies themselves that Rose described in the 1980s.[36] In relation to sex, rights have come to be attached to the freedom to have sex; not to the freedom to love whom one chooses, but to the freedom to choose itself. This makes it very difficult in Western liberal societies to appeal to the common good. But even these societies contain within them active traditions which emphasize interdependence. The philosopher Charles Taylor has argued that even individualism, as a moral ideal, must offer a view on how one should live with others.[37] He argues that choice only matters against a horizon of value that is in relation to some view of the good.

Implications

It is clear that our understanding about sex and sexually-transmitted infections should include the fact that some behaviours 'raise the burden and effects of disease for all'.[38] And the evidence is that in certain situations that understanding will affect the behaviour of people in ways that will reduce HIV prevalence in the society.[39] Education, aimed at enhancing understanding and hence the will of the individual, has an accepted moral mandate in public health.[40] There is also a specific moral dimension that is related to the meaning of sexual relationships. The call to avoid affecting the level of disease in the commons gets its moral force partly from care for the other within a sexual relationship. A pamphlet published in New York in the early days of the AIDS epidemic questioned the wisdom of encouraging the separation of love and affection from sex and suggested that keeping affection alive might be a crucial motive for protecting a sexual partner and the community.[41] This of course takes us back to making moral distinctions—that sex within a meaningful relationship is better than outside it. Then the crucial issue is whether this position can be held without undermining another important value: that people should not be judged because of their sexual behaviour?

---

[36] Rose, *Strategy of Preventive Medicine*.

[37] C. Taylor, *The Ethics of Authenticity* (Cambridge MA: Harvard University Press, 1991).

[38] Shelton et al., 'Parter reduction is crucial'.

[39] Stoneburner & Low-Beer, 'Population-level HIV declines'.

[40] P. Cole, 'The moral bases for public health interventions', in L.O. Goslin (ed.) *Public Health Law and Ethics: a Reader* (Berkeley, CA: University of California Press, 2002).

[41] 'How to have sex in an epidemic: one approach', *News from the Front* (NY: 1983).

The difficulties with this approach are legion. But the growing call for an end to polarizing debate on HIV prevention methods,[42] the challenge to address sexual ethics around HIV prevention in a less morally cramped fashion,[43] and the increasing attention to the cultural context in which HIV transmission takes place[44] might allow these moral dimensions to re-enter the conversation.

---

42 D.T. Halperin, M.J. Sleiner, M.M. Cassell, et al., 'The time has come for common ground on preventing sexual transmission of HIV', *Lancet*, 364 (2004): 1913-14.

43 R. Bayer, 'AIDS prevention-sexual ethics and responsibility', *New England Journal of Medicine*, 334 (1996): 1540-42.

44 Poundstone et al., 'The social epidemiology'.

Chapter 16

Contagious Disease and Rights

T.M. Wilkinson

Auckland University, New Zealand

Put at its starkest, it seems you can have rights or public health, but not both. At least, this seems so as far as preventing the spread of contagious disease is concerned. On the one hand, innocent people have rights not to be restricted in their freedom of movement and association, and yet quarantine (separation of those exposed to disease) and isolation (separation of those with symptoms) do precisely that. They have rights to bodily integrity, which are surely compromised by compulsory vaccination or compulsory medical tests and treatments; and they have rights to medical confidentiality, and yet these seem breached when public health officers or close contacts, including sexual partners, are informed without the consent of rightholders. On the other hand, these infringements of rights might prevent untold misery and death from tuberculosis, SARS, HIV/AIDS, smallpox, avian flu or any of a whole host of old or emerging terrible diseases. Hence the apparent conflict between rights and public health.

Perhaps conflict between rights and public health could be avoided if, with the right infrastructure and communication, people would willingly comply with the instructions of public health officials. Perhaps compulsion is unnecessary because sick people are unable to act against those instructions. Perhaps compulsion would backfire because people will resist, stay away from medical treatment, or fail to comply with instructions. Some believe, for these reasons, that compulsion is very rarely required to control contagious disease, while others claim that compulsion is a useful extra tool.[1] If compulsion were needed to do some good, the apparent conflict with rights raises the questions of whether and why public health powers would be ethically-justified. This is a venerable problem, but not one that has attracted much sophisticated philosophical discussion. A recent slew of articles speculate about why public health ethics in general is neglected,[2] and I shall not

---

[1] See the exchange between two leading writers in the field. L.O. Gostin defends compulsion in 'When Terrorism Threatens Health: How Far are Limitations on Personal and Economic Liberties Justified?', *Florida Law Review*, 55/5 (2003) and he is criticized in the same issue by G. Annas, `Puppy Love: Bioterrorism, Civil Rights, and Public Health'. See also Gostin's book-length discussion, *Public Health Law: Power*, *Duty*, *Restraint* (Berkeley and Los Angeles: University of California Press, 2000).

[2] See e.g. M.J. Selgelid, 'Ethics and Infectious Disease' *Bioethics* 19/3 (2005); L. Francis, M. Battin, J. Jacobson, C. Smith and J. Botkin, 'How Infectious Diseases Got

speculate further here. The aim of this chapter is to provide a rough map, from within a framework of rights, of some ways to think through the problem.

Assume that people ordinarily have personal rights, such as rights to bodily integrity, freedom of movement and association, and confidentiality. Let 'compulsion' be the loose shorthand term for the putative infringements of rights. Compulsion for the sake of controlling contagious disease might be justified on the grounds that while these rights are important, they are not absolute, and when there is enough good, they may be overridden. Or it might be that people do not have rights against compulsion when it is needed to defend other people's rights against being infected—an idea of self-defence. Lastly, it might be that the collective action problems created by contagious disease justify compulsion. This chapter explores each of these ideas of overriding rights, self-defence, and collective action problems. As we think through each, we find different accounts of the scope and limits of justified public health compulsion. It should be said that, when it comes to the details, none of these ideas is straightforward or uncontroversial, as I shall indicate as we go through. The map offered here is both rough and an indicator of future lines of research.

Overriding People's Rights To Do Good

Even those who usually reject compulsion in public health do not argue that the rights we are considering, such as the right to refuse medical treatment or to guarantee confidentiality, are absolute, that is, rights it would be wrong to infringe upon no matter what the consequences. Their objection is that the restrictions do not work, not that they infringe on absolute rights.[3] If the rights are not absolute, then it is in principle permissible to infringe on them. If the rights may be infringed on, then when and why? An obvious initial answer is: when it would do enough good or, what I shall take as equivalent, averting enough harm. But how much good must there be to override a right?

Many utilitarians and other consequentialists would say that, leaving aside side-effects on trust and other such considerations, rights may be infringed on even for the sake of the tiniest bit of net gain.[4] Non-consequentialists say that the compulsion that infringes on a right would have to do a significantly greater

---

Left Out—and What This Omission Might Have Meant For Bioethics', *Bioethics*, 19/4 (2005).

[3] Annas, 'Puppy Love', p. 1179.

[4] E.g. S. Kagan, *The Limits of Morality* (Oxford: Oxford University Press, 1989), Chapters 3 and 4. Utilitarians might also say that we should not leave aside side-effects, and in practice their view, like the non-consequentialist view, might recommend extra weight for rights. See R.M. Hare, *Moral Thinking* (Oxford: Oxford University Press, 1981): pp. 132-5.

amount of good than the loss the rightholder suffers.[5] Let us set the controversy aside and say that the infringement of a right is justified only if it produces an amount of good above some threshold, leaving it open how far above the loss to the rightholder this threshold must be. Where this threshold lies also depends on the rights in question. Breaking into your car might be justified to get someone to hospital but breaking into you might not be. At least part of the reason why is that infringing on some rights tends to cause more harm to the rightholder than infringing on others. Harm might not be the only consideration but, other things equal, the more harm that rightholders would suffer, the more good would have to be done as a result of infringing on their rights.[6] This claim that harm determines thresholds supports several intuitive judgements we might make about public health cases.

Consider the famous US Supreme Court case of *Jacobson v. Massachusetts* (1905).[7] Henning Jacobson argued against being held liable for refusing a smallpox vaccination under a Cambridge, Massachusetts law requiring this of adults. One of Jacobson's arguments was that he was especially prone to an adverse reaction to the vaccination. While the Court did not accept that Jacobson had shown himself sufficiently sensitive to win exemption, they did accept that, in principle, those who were especially susceptible to severe reactions should not be forced to be vaccinated. The view that harm determines thresholds can justify this intuitively plausible judgement. Special susceptibility means a likelihood of suffering extra harm, and so it would take further good, in the case of the especially susceptible, to justify infringing on their rights to refuse vaccinations than it would to justify infringing on the rights of the less susceptible. On the assumption that there would not be that much good from forcibly vaccinating the susceptible, the susceptible should not be forced.

The state can compel in more or less severe forms. Intuitively, it takes more good to justify the more severe compulsion and, again, this can be explained by the view that the more harm a rightholder would suffer through infringement, the more good must be done. In *Jacobson*, the penalty for non-compliance was only a $5 fine. However, states have prevented children from attending school without being vaccinated, which is more serious. In emergencies, the state could threaten to imprison people or force them at gunpoint, or threaten to separate parents from

---

5 Unfortunately, and rather unsatisfactorily, it is not possible to be exact about how much more, given the current state of the non-consequentialist art in moral and political philosophy, S. Brennan, 'Thresholds for Rights', *The Southern Journal of Philosophy*, 33 (1995): 146; S. Kagan, *Normative Ethics* (Boulder: Westview, 1998): pp. 311-12.

6 S. Brennan, 'How Is the Strength of a Right Determined?', *American Philosophical Quarterly*, 32 (1995); J.J. Thomson, *The Realm of Rights* (Cambridge MA: Harvard University Press, 1990): Chapter 6.

7 The judgement is excerpted in L.O.Gostin, *Public Health Law and Ethics: A Reader*, (Berkeley and Los Angeles: University of California Press, 2002): pp. 206-15.

their children.[8] Suffering a $5 fine, even at 1905 prices, is one thing; having one's children removed is an altogether more serious harm. It might then be that, for any given amount of good, while some forms of compulsion would be permissible, others would not, even if they were necessary to achieve that good. It might not be permissible to secure higher vaccination rates by breaking up the families of those who refuse, even if that were the only way to get the higher rates.

The idea we are considering is that rights may be overridden when it would do enough good. However, the amount of good that compulsion would do is a matter of probability. Carriers of disease might not infect anyone or they might infect many, who might then infect others. The negativity of being infected is also a matter of probability. When people fail to complete a course of treatment for tuberculosis, the disease has a probability of reactivating and developing into a multi-drug resistant strain, so people might catch a strain that is easier or harder to treat.[9] Some diseases, like polio, kill some people and cause severe disability in others, but produce only minor symptoms in the vast majority of cases.[10] Thus to be set against the infringement of an individual's right is a probability mix of nothing happening, some being infected, and many being infected, along with probabilities for the severity of the effects of the disease. That an infringement would only probably achieve some good does not mean that the infringement must be unjustified. It is surely correct to say that, if rights are not absolute, they may be overridden to prevent probable harm, for at least harms and probabilities above some level. There is, however, further work to be done in establishing that level.

Overriding rights is permissible only if enough good is done, and we have seen some of the complications in setting thresholds and taking account of probabilities. There are further questions that a developed view of overriding rights would have to deal with. Compulsory measures, for instance, medical treatment or vaccination, might benefit those whose rights are infringed upon. One tricky question is about the extent to which these benefits would justify the infringement.[11] Another is about the total good. Clearly, the more people who could be protected from disease by a restriction, the more reason there would be to restrict. But should the total benefit consist of an aggregation of all benefits, small and large? If so, it is in principle possible that quarantining someone with a cold could be justified, if it would prevent a large enough number of colds to others, but this seems counter-intuitive. Or does averting only serious harms count for the total good? These

---

[8] This was the fear of the Association of American Physicians and Surgeons in their comment on Florida's law-giving powers to force treatment on the unwilling. See Annas, 'Puppy Love', p. 1186.

[9] R. Bayer and A.L. Fairchild, 'The Genesis of Public Health Ethics', *Bioethics*, 18/6 (2004): 489.

[10] G.N. Grob, *The Deadly Truth: A History of Disease in America* (Cambridge MA: Harvard University Press, 2002): p. 189.

[11] S. Brennan, 'Paternalism and Rights', *Canadian Journal of Philosophy*, 24 (1994).

questions shall have to be left aside here, with the closing comment that overriding rights is not as straightforward an idea as it might at first appear.

Self-Defence[12]

Overriding rights is not the only way to think of justifying public health compulsion, nor the best for a range of cases. Consider people who intentionally, recklessly, or negligently endanger the health of others. People who would deliberately infect salad bars with salmonella, wave syringes with HIV-positive blood in a shopping mall, or engage in unprotected intercourse while keeping information about their sexually-transmitted infections to themselves, do not have a right to do any of these things and are infringing on the rights of others not to be infected. So if some compulsory measure stops them, it seems misleading to say that their rights have been overridden, as though they were innocents being sacrificed for the greater good. Rather, the justification for compulsion seems to lie within the principles of self- and other-defence.

There are important differences between saying 'public health compulsion is justified for the sake of the overall good' and 'public health compulsion is justified in self-defence'. If compulsion is to be a justified overriding of rights, most views of rights say that it would take a lot of extra good to justify the harm to the rightholder. This might make compulsion wrong in many cases. However, if compulsion can be justified as self-defence, much changes. If someone is about to attack and seriously injure me, I may in self-defence use deadly force. In general, self-defence allows us to do more harm, to the threat, than good, to us. If compulsion is a form of legitimate self-defence, then it would take a lot less to justify it than if it is simply overriding rights for the sake of more good.

A second difference between overriding and self-defence is in entitlements to compensation. It is widely taken that to infringe upon people's rights is to wrong them and to owe compensation. Even if a person's right is permissibly infringed upon, to prevent great social harm for instance, it does not disappear. One of the 'traces' the right leaves is an obligation on those infringing to compensate the rightholder.[13] In this example, compensation is not morally optional. But in the cases of the salad bar, syringe, and sex, and unlike a case where a person's rights are sacrificed for the sake of the greater good, we do not have a sense that the people are owed compensation for not being allowed to endanger others.

Suppose we accept that the intentional, reckless and negligent may be acted against in self-defence. There is still some way to go to defend public health compulsion, which is not private self-defence. But it is widely accepted, and

[12] There is much more detail on this in my 'Contagious Disease and Self-Defence', *Res Publica*, 13/4 (2007): 339-59.

[13] Thomson stresses this point in several places in *Realm of Rights* and *Rights, Restitution and Risk* (Cambridge MA: Harvard University Press, 1986).

seems unproblematic to claim, that the principles that underlie self-defence can justify defending others from threats, and so can justify the collective action of a public health service.[14] Any compulsion would be subject to traditional constraints on self-defence, such as proportionality and minimum force, but let us put these to one side. There is then a question about the scope of a justification of self-defence. It includes those at fault, but what about those people who are not responsible for being threats? And how large is the category of the non-responsible?

First, the question of self-defence against the non-responsible. Some people would be non-responsible threats because, in short, they do not know what they are doing. This would include small children and those with certain kinds of mental illness or disability. From some viewpoints one could justify restrictions against the non-responsible on the grounds of self-defence, and on others, one could not.[15] This is another of those controversies that I shall have to indicate and then pass on. Now I move on to the question of the size of the category of the non-responsible.

Let us take it that many people with contagious diseases are not responsible for their conditions. They might nonetheless be responsible for being threats to the health of others. They would be responsible if they were credibly told that they were a threat and told how they could avoid being threats. Suppose the public health service has done just this. If the contagious then refuse to act as advised, they seem to become responsible threats, not non-responsible threats. They would then be liable to be acted against in self-defence. This suggests that the scope of a self-defence justification is not limited to those responsible for acquiring their diseases.

In addition to responsibility, there is a further question about the threats against which self-defence can be justified. May we act against suspected threats and, if so, on the basis of what suspicions? Measures like compulsory quarantine, screening and vaccination look problematic once this question is asked. These measures predictably include people who do not and would not threaten others. To be sure, they will also catch genuine threats and the reason for catching the others is that threats are not clearly identifiable. But people are constrained in how they may respond in self-defence to an unidentifiable threat. Suppose, firstly, that an assassin with a moderately good aim is coming for me in a crowd of 200 people. I cannot legitimately imprison the whole crowd in self-defence, even if that is the only way to protect myself. The other 199 have not done anything to threaten me. By parallel, one might conclude that one may not lock down an apartment complex of 200 people known to contain one person infected with SARS. The other 199 have also done nothing to threaten me. The general point is that people who do not causally threaten others because they are not infected are innocent bystanders and if they were compelled into quarantine, vaccination, or screening, their rights would be

---

14 J.J. Thomson, 'Self-Defense', *Philosophy and Public Affairs*, 20/4 (1991): 283-310.

15 R. Nozick, *Anarchy, State, and Utopia* (Oxford: Oxford University Press, 1974): p.34; Thomson, *Realm of Rights*, p. 336f.; J. McMahan, *The Ethics of Killing* (New York: Oxford University Press, 2002): p. 398f.

infringed upon. Compelling nonetheless may be permissible, as the section on overriding rights pointed out, but it would not be legitimate self-defence.

This section has considered a self-defence justification of public health restrictions. The contrast with the previous section, on overriding rights, is that restrictions need do less good to be justified if they are legitimate self-defence than if they override rights. There are, though, questions about when and whether public health compulsion is legitimate self-defence. While I avoided the question of compelling the non-responsible, I did claim that the category of the responsible was larger than one might think, since it does not exclude those who are not responsible for acquiring their conditions. However, there are occasions when public health compulsion is harder to justify in self-defence, and an instance of the application of quarantine was given as one example.

Waiving Rights and the Problems of Individual Cooperation

So far, public health compulsion has been described as doing bad, or at least unwanted, things to some people for the sake of preventing bad things happening to others. This is somewhat misleading because many people would welcome a regime of public health compulsion, judging that the expected gains to them outweigh the costs they expect to pay. But why would they need to be compelled? The argument here builds on the idea that individual action can produce collectively bad (and individually-regretted) results.

Vaccination and herd protection is often discussed as a prime example in public health of a case where the maximal pursuit of individual self-interest has bad results for each individual. If enough people get vaccinated, some diseases can no longer survive—the herd is protected. Herd protection is of benefit to everyone, not just those who have been vaccinated. Being vaccinated is a cost. In this analysis, each prefers not to vaccinate if others do, and attempts to freeride on others, getting the benefit of herd protection without running any of the risks of vaccination. But if each acts on this preference, there is no herd protection and all are worse off even in terms of their own preferences.[16] This analysis works just as well when we take account of the fact that many decisions about vaccinations are made by parents about their children. The point that free and not irrational individual action can make individuals worse off is, however, more general than vaccination and applies to contagious disease as a whole.

In a significant recent article, Richard Epstein defends traditional compulsion in public health, including quarantine and vaccination, by using a thought experiment

[16] T. Dare, 'Mass Immunisation Programmes: Some Philosophical Issues', *Bioethics*, 12 (1998): 137; A. Dawson, 'Vaccination and the Prevention Problem', *Bioethics*, 18/6 (2004): 515-30. Both authors are much more careful in how they handle this problem than this short account can show.

to show the failures of a *laissez faire* model.[17] In this model, people have rights over their bodies and tort law protects them against wrongful harm through *ex ante* injunction and *ex post* compensation. Epstein argues that these protections are inadequate against contagious disease. Even assuming people who infect others should be liable, for some diseases we are all potential infectors or infected and we cannot all take out injunctions against each other. Nor can we reliably expect compensation from those who infect us, since we will probably not know who they are, or else they would not be in any state to pay.

Epstein then writes, 'Some (but not all) forms of direct regulation hold out the possibility of increasing security for all at the expense of liberty. So long as each regards himself as the gainer from this massive social exchange, who should protest about it in the abstract?'.[18] And then, subject to certain conditions, 'The basic *laissez-faire* account of police power holds: everyone is a net gainer from behind the veil of ignorance of the uniform application of quarantine rules'.[19] (By the 'veil of ignorance' I take it that he means: people do not know at the time of choice whether they will actually be subject to quarantine or saved by quarantine from infection.) There have to be rules accepted in advance. Free choice later on would have some people breaking quarantine, not getting vaccinated, and so on, producing results that all do or can agree in advance are worse than those produced by compulsion.

Epstein's claims are worth exploring rather further than he does in his article. If they can persuade even those generally opposed to state action, they might persuade everyone. One way to move from premises about the collectively bad results of individual action to a conclusion in favour of compulsion is via consequentialist considerations: there would be more good achieved with compulsion than without. But this misses the point of Epstein's justifications, which focus on the benefits to the individuals who are compelled. It is not that some are sacrificed for the sake of greater benefits to others; it is that each stands to benefit from compulsion. However, there are two different ways to take the justification. Epstein's first version says 'so long as *each regards himself as the gainer*' [italics added] which locates the justification in the attitude of people towards the benefits; the second says 'everyone is a net gainer' which locates the justification in the actual benefits. These are significantly different. Since people might benefit without thinking they do, or believe they benefit even when they do not, these justifications can come apart.

Suppose, as in Epstein's thought experiment, 'each regards himself as the gainer'. Why would this make it permissible later to compel people? It could be that, while people do have rights not to be compelled, they have waived these rights in advance in order to secure the benefits of a regime of compulsion. People prefer health to a general refusal to comply and would give up a right to refuse

---

[17] R. Epstein, 'Let the Shoemaker Stick to His Last: A Defense of the "Old" Public Health', *Perspectives in Biology and Medicine*, 46/3 (2003): S138-59.

[18] Ibid., p. 143.

[19] Ibid., p. 145.

if they could be sure of people generally giving up their rights. This is a form of hypothetical consent, and it is a matter of controversy how much force hypothetical consent has. Let us say that rights count as waived where rightholders do, or would if asked, endorse the compulsion and waive their rights against it. With further polishing and specification, and bracketing the controversy about hypothetical consent, this is potentially a powerful argument for public health compulsion. (It also goes beyond anything Epstein says in his article.)

The drawback for the waiving argument is that it is probably not true that all would regard themselves as gainers from compulsory measures. There are indefinitely many types of restrictions that could be adopted: so much of setting a certain judicial hurdle before breaching confidentiality; allowing compulsory quarantine on breaths of suspicion or only with solid evidence; keeping even close family away from the sick and dying, or permitting that contact but preventing others, and so on. For all, or all but the most minimal, it is overwhelmingly likely that not everyone would prospectively consent. In a word, some holdouts would reject regimes of compulsion that even a large majority might favour. A similar problem applies to the specific case of vaccination; not everyone who refuses to vaccinate is trying to freeride. Some genuinely think the vaccination immoral or harmful. In a system with mandatory vaccination, they would not regard themselves as the gainers. Because, from the viewpoint given here, waiving a right requires that the rightholder actually agrees, or at least endorses the compulsion, and because holdouts neither endorse nor agree, the holdouts have not waived their rights.

The second justification says that what counts are the actual benefits, not people's attitudes to them. To continue with vaccination, supposing mandatory near-universal vaccination would so reduce disease that everyone would benefit compared with the level of vaccination achieved through individual free choice, even when one takes into account the moral and other costs of compulsion, how does this assumed fact justify compelling the non-believers? There could be a straightforwardly paternalistic argument: vaccination is so good for people, they should be forced into it. Obviously, paternalism, toward competent adults anyway, is highly controversial. Or it could be a fairness or reciprocity argument: people have received the benefits and they should pay for them. But this is also controversial.[20] People do not have to pay for philosophy lectures they have not asked for even if they benefit from them, so why should they, on grounds of fairness or reciprocity, have to contribute to a public good they neither recognize nor want?[21]

Where people do willingly accept the benefits of public health compulsion, they may be made to comply either because they have waived their rights not to or because of fairness, or both. That is the positive conclusion of this section, and it adds to the stock of defences of public health compulsion so far given. There is

---

20 A. John Simmons, *On the Edge of Anarchy* (Princeton NJ: Princeton University Press, 1993): pp. 249-61. See also Dare, 'Mass Immunisation', pp. 144-8.

21 Nozick, *Anarchy*, p. 93f.

also a negative conclusion: where people do not willingly accept the benefits, they still have rights not to comply, with anything that has been said in this section.

Conclusion

This chapter has set out a framework for assessing the ethics of public health restrictions from the perspective of rights. It has described three ways to justify public health restrictions. One is to say that the rights are overridden by the good that the restrictions would do. Another is to say that the restrictions are a legitimate form of self-defence. A third is to regard people as having waived their rights. All of these ideas need, and are worth, further development. As a rough statement, though, we can say that a restriction is justified if it is a justified overriding of rights or legitimate self-defence or a restriction against which people have waived their rights. We can also say that, if a restriction is none of these things, it is not justified since, by hypothesis, it is not legitimate self-defence and it conflicts with people's rights, which are not justifiably overridden or waived.

These justifications have their own interest in helping us work out whether and when public health compulsion would be ethically permissible. They also support this conclusion about how we should interpret the ethical problem of compulsion: we should be careful before seeing it as a conflict between rights and public health. This is partly because of well-aired doubts about the usefulness of compulsion in controlling contagious disease. But it is also for less-well-aired philosophical points about rights.[22]

[22] An earlier version was given at the School of Public Health, the University of Texas at Houston, and a conference at the School of Population Health, the University of Auckland. My thanks to the audiences for their comments, and also to Julian Lamont and Andrew Moore.

Index